Praise for
Advancing Reproductive Choice

~

"Liz Maguire looks back at a brilliant career and noble mission to show the way forward. Her passionate memoir will be an inspiration for the new generation of leaders to advance reproductive choice for all. They can make a difference following her role model of leadership with conviction and compassion."

—MAHMOUD F. FATHALLA, MD, PhD, former President of the International Federation of Gynecology and Obstetrics

"Liz Maguire is one of the most passionate, determined, and humble people I have ever met, and I am lucky to call her my mentor. Her memoir provides a rich and unique perspective into the journey of an unwavering and compassionate leader in the sexual and reproductive health and rights (SRHR) field. In her book, Liz grapples with completing the unfinished agenda to realize SRHR for all. As I look ahead, I see a bright future where young and seasoned leaders work together to shift inequitable power structures that hold young women back from leading. In this future I envision, all leaders can learn from one another and ultimately grow together as they fight for SRHR, just as Liz and I have done."

—ANA AGUILERA, MPH, Deputy Director of Adolescent and Youth Sexual and Reproductive Health, EngenderHealth

"How absolutely brilliant and truly exhilarating. I love *Advancing Reproductive Choice: Leading with Conviction and Compassion!* This memoir is a true and ardent record of the quest for the reproductive health and rights of women everywhere but especially and urgently for the deprived women in poor countries. It is a chronicle of a life well lived in the service of country, of women, and of the world, with helpful insights on core values and leadership. BRAVO."

—AMBASSADOR DR. EUNICE BROOKMAN-AMISSAH, MB.ChB, FWACP.FRCOG, former Ipas Vice President for Africa

"At its core, *Advancing Reproductive Choice* is a moving story of unwavering personal commitment, continuous innovation, and engagement of a broad spectrum of leaders and activists in the pursuit of advancing sexual and reproductive health and rights for all. Liz Maguire embodies the axiom 'the personal is political' and grounds her vision in the understanding that all women have the right to choose the reproductive options that make the most sense in their lives. This book covers a critical historical period of important gains and ongoing challenges to the idea that self-determination and abortion access are a critical element of women's rights. It is an essential read for all those interested in reproductive rights and justice."

—LEILA HESSINI, MA, MPH, Vice President, Programs,
Global Fund for Women

"Liz Maguire's memoir goes beyond being a chronicle of an amazing 45-year career as a global influencer of sexual and reproductive health and rights, to a valuable guide for anyone interested in public health, values-centered leadership, or maximizing life's opportunities. Her considerable knowledge and leadership experience make this book a must-read for young professionals starting their career in development, managers wanting to transform to values-centered leadership, and just about anyone wanting to design a life they love."

—VINOJ MANNING, MBA, Chief Executive Officer,
Ipas Development Foundation, India

"We revel in the benefits of great leadership, appreciating them only after losing them to change. In this memoir of her remarkable international career, Liz Maguire generously shares her wisdom from leading mission-focused organizations with passion and compassion. If you are a friend or relative, enjoy her lifestyle guidance on travel, nutrition, music, and reading. If you are a young girl, adolescent, or woman, thank her profusely for enabling your life's reproductive choices."

—AMY TSUI, PhD, Professor Emerita, Bloomberg School of
Public Health, Johns Hopkins University

Advancing Reproductive Choice

Advancing Reproductive Choice

～

Leading with Conviction
and Compassion

A MEMOIR

ELIZABETH S. MAGUIRE

MONT BORON PRESS
Chapel Hill, North Carolina, USA
Nice, France

Advancing Reproductive Choice
by Elizabeth S. Maguire
MONT BORON PRESS
Chapel Hill, North Carolina | Nice, France
advancingreproductivechoice.org
To contact the author: maguire@advancingreproductivechoice.org

© 2020 Elizabeth S. Maguire
All rights reserved. No part of this publication may be reproduced, stored in a
retrieval system, or transmitted, in any form or in any means—electronic,
mechanical, photocopying, recording, or otherwise—without prior permission,
except as permitted by U.S. copyright law.

Editor: Karen Barrett-Wilt
Book and cover design: Sara DeHaan
Map: DNCmaps.com | Madison, WI

Photo credits: All photos are by the author or are her property except where
otherwise credited. Cover: Visiting Corporation Hospital in Aurangabad, India, 2013.
© Ipas Development Foundation (IDF)

Publisher's Cataloging-in-Publication Data

Names: Maguire, Elizabeth S., author.
Title: Advancing reproductive choice : leading with conviction and compassion ,
a memoir / Elizabeth S. Maguire.
Description: Chapel Hill, NC; Nice, France: Mont Boron Press, 2020.
Identifiers: LCCN: 2020912037 | ISBN: 978-0-578-73391-3 (pbk.) |
978-0-578-73392-0 (ebook)
Subjects: LCSH Maguire, Elizabeth S. | Maguire, Elizabeth S.—Travel—Developing
countries. | Maguire, Elizabeth S.—Travel—Europe. | Reproductive rights—
History—20th century. | Reproductive rights—21st century. | Women—Health and
hygiene—Developing countries. | Reproductive health services. | Contraception—
Developing countries. | Sexual health—Developing countries. | United States. Agency
for International Development—Officials and employees—Biography. | Leadership. |
Mentorship. | BISAC BIOGRAPHY & AUTOBIOGRAPHY / Personal Memoirs | SOCIAL
SCIENCE / Abortion and Birth Control | BUSINESS & ECONOMICS / Leadership
Classification: LCC RG136.M34 2020 | DDC 613.9/092—dc23

To everyone engaged in the global fight for sexual and reproductive health and rights and for gender equality,

To all who demand racial and economic justice in the U.S. and around the world,

and

To frontline heroes during the COVID-19 pandemic and those who have suffered the loss of loved ones and livelihoods

CONTENTS

Introduction

What counts in life is not the mere fact that we have lived. It is what difference we have made to the lives of others that will determine the significance of the life we lead.

—Nelson Mandela

From a distance, I saw a young woman lying on the ground in tremendous pain and hemorrhaging badly. The other sick people near her were also waiting to get into the hospital but were accompanied by family members. There were no health care providers in sight; they were attending to other patients inside the crowded facility in Dakar, Senegal. It was heartbreaking to witness this teenager all alone, with no one comforting her or trying to save her life. I learned later from a nurse that the young woman died as a result of sepsis from a self-induced or back-alley abortion. Her tragic death could have been prevented if she had received the information and quality care she deserved.

Forty-eight years later, this image is still vivid in my mind. Sadly, this experience remains a common occurrence throughout Africa, Asia, and Latin America. Even with all the advances in health care and technologies over the last half-century, each year there are well over 22,800 women who die from unsafe abortions. Another seven million are hospitalized, many with serious injuries. More than 214 million women want to avoid a pregnancy but are not using a modern method of contraception. These estimates will increase dramatically as a result of the COVID-19 pandemic.

Watching the young Senegalese woman suffer such a lonely and senseless death during my first trip to Africa in 1972 had a profound impact. It was a key motivating factor in my pursuing a career where I could contribute to saving and improving women's lives in the developing world.

In every country, there are countless unsung heroes together with well-known leaders who have devoted their lives to helping women and girls exercise their fundamental human right: to safely prevent and manage unwanted pregnancies. I applaud and am humbled by the tremendous dedication and efforts of all these individuals. I hope my story *Advancing*

Reproductive Choice: Leading with Conviction and Compassion will nevertheless offer elements of interest and inspiration to others, especially to those who have embraced this critical cause.

I highlight in this memoir many of the rich experiences I have had and the extraordinary people I have met around the world. I have been deeply moved by the suffering and resilience of poor women and girls in every region. At the same time, I have been impressed by the commitment of health care providers and visionary leaders to enhance the well-being of all people.

In my book, I discuss the unique role and impact of the organizations where I have worked, focusing on the years I spent at each one. I hope I have faithfully portrayed, to the best of my recollection, some of the key events and accomplishments, reflecting the contributions of my many colleagues who inspired me.

Together, we have witnessed enormous changes. We participated in the paradigm shift from an initial emphasis on family planning to a broader focus, in the early 1990s, on the sexual and reproductive health and rights (SRHR) of women and girls. More recently, attention has turned to the needs of individuals of all sexual identities. Gender-based violence and gender equality, along with women's empowerment, are receiving heightened priority. However, moving from rhetoric to lasting change is a long process. It requires greatly increased commitment, action, and resources.

Since the 1970s, it has been encouraging to see a significant expansion in the number of women and adolescents accessing modern contraceptive methods and other reproductive health services, including safe, legal abortions. But these gains have fallen far short of meeting all the needs, especially as we assess the full impact of the global coronavirus pandemic. Along with improvements in the quality, accessibility, and affordability of these vital services, there have been setbacks in many countries, including in the U.S. Those who are suffering the most are young people, urban and rural poor, displaced persons, refugees, and other vulnerable populations. In this book, I offer reflections on global progress to date, the huge unmet needs, and the long road ahead in ensuring sexual and reproductive health and rights for all. Tragically, these challenges have been greatly exacerbated by the novel coronavirus. The human and economic toll from this global disaster is staggering and continues to escalate.

Now in my retirement years, I have transitioned from being a CEO to a focus on "giving back" and making the most of life's opportunities. Despite dealing with some health issues, the period of confinement, and the death of several friends from COVID-19, I have tried to maintain a positive spirit. These periods, however painful, provide time for reflection and personal growth.

We can all look back at key moments in our lives, the choices we have made, and what we might have done differently if given another chance. I believe we must learn from our mistakes, keep moving forward, and open new chapters. We must cherish those close to us, express appreciation, help those in need, and live life to the fullest, no matter what difficulties may be present.

During the last few years, my husband, Terry, and I have enjoyed spending more time with family and friends both in the U.S. and in France, our second home. Since retiring, we have been living up to six months a year on the other side of the Atlantic, experiencing many adventures and rewarding moments. This will change, at least in the immediate future, as a result of social distancing and travel restrictions due to COVID-19. During this unprecedented time, I am grateful to be able to pursue my wide-ranging interests and contribute to my number one passion: advancing sexual and reproductive health and rights around the world.

In this memoir, I reflect on the core values that have guided me throughout my life and the lessons I have learned. The key principles I highlight are passion, empowerment, and perseverance, along with compassion, love and friendship, and gratitude. Among my other guiding principles are enthusiasm, optimism, kindness, humility, curiosity, and continuous learning. Living core values is paramount in whatever path you choose in life and in helping others achieve their goals as well. We can all appreciate the importance of core values as we witness the widespread suffering and loss on a scale unparalleled in our lifetime. Moreover, we must adjust to significant changes in how we live, work, and interact with others.

Effective leadership, especially during times of crisis, is essential across all sectors and at all levels. I share thoughts on leadership from my experience in government and with international non-profit organizations where I was fortunate to hold positions of responsibility for over four decades. I comment on what I consider are fundamental personal characteristics of leaders. Many of these qualities are more commonly associated with women in positions of power. Since I began my career, I have seen a revolution in the workplace—from one dominated by men who held almost all the leadership positions to one where women are playing vital roles. Indeed, women are making transformative contributions in my field and others. But they must be given the same opportunities, recognition, and compensation as men.

Major gender inequities continue to exist in the U.S. and in every country around the globe. Fighting for the fundamental rights of women and girls, and for people of all gender identities—from control over their bodies to equity in all aspects of life—is an ongoing battle. What is needed is the vision, dedication, and full engagement of leaders and activists everywhere.

Some of the most gratifying experiences I have had throughout my career and in retirement are supporting and mentoring young leaders, mostly women, from every region. They have wanted to know more about how I chose my profession, key pathways, and milestones, and my most exciting as well as difficult moments. Their questions have focused on how to advance in their lives and careers, make the most of opportunities, and deal effectively with setbacks. Most of all, they have been anxious to talk about how to be great leaders, inspiring and motivating others. These young people have shared their hopes and dreams as well as their creative ideas. I have been energized by their enthusiasm and desire to make a difference in the lives of others.

I have learned a lot from interacting with these rising stars as well as with other leaders in different stages of their careers. I hope that I have helped some of them, even to a small degree, in their journeys. I believe that the young leaders of today and tomorrow are pivotal to accelerating progress in solving the world's most intractable problems and inequities, including in the area of women's fundamental human rights.

This book is a salute to all who have fought for or are currently carrying the torch for a healthier, more just, and peaceful world. It is also a tribute to everyone who has enriched my life.

PART ONE

BEGINNING MY JOURNEY

DEFINING MOMENTS AND NEW HORIZONS

1

Gifts from My Family

Our lives are defined by pivotal moments and turning points. With the support of a loving family, I had the chance to follow my passions. These opportunities opened new horizons as I moved through my childhood into adulthood and found my partner and mission in life.

I was blessed to grow up in a warm, close-knit family with parents who instilled in their children core values of love, compassion, humility, kindness, and service to others. They emphasized the importance of studying, working hard, and leading a purposeful life. From a young age, I also had a strong independent spirit coupled with a desire to "push the boundaries" and "explore new frontiers."

My parents and grandparents provided a solid spiritual and intellectual framework for us along with the hope that our lives would be happy and fulfilling. My paternal grandfather, Henry H. Shires, was an extraordinary individual on many dimensions. Despite coming from a family of very modest means, he graduated from Cornell University with a degree in electrical engineering and then attended General Theological Seminary in New York City to become an Episcopal minister. Following several years of a long-distance courtship, he married my grandmother (Mable Millis), an accomplished singer.

Soon after the birth of their son in 1913, my grandfather decided to move the family to Arizona. He left behind a wealthy community in New Jersey to do missionary work in what was then the "Wild West." Much of his time he spent on horseback travelling to different communities, preaching, and caring for the sick and dying. My grandmother slept with a gun under her pillow at night because they lived in a mining area where it was not safe to leave the house in the evening. In 1918, the family moved to northern California, settling in the San Francisco Bay area. There, my grandfather served as Rector of Christ Episcopal Church in Alameda for 17 years. For the following 15 years, he was Dean of the Church Divinity School of the Pacific, a graduate school in Berkeley providing advanced degrees in Divinity. In 1950, Dean Shires was elected the first Suffragan Bishop of the Episcopal Church in California, a post he held for eight years. His sudden death in 1961 from a heart attack was a great loss to all who admired Bishop Shires for his leadership, caring, charisma, and wit.

While I only knew my paternal grandfather until I turned 14, I have rich and loving memories of him. He left a major imprint on all the people he touched during his life. He had a magnetic personality and a twinkle in his eye. "Ga-um," as my sister and I called him from the time

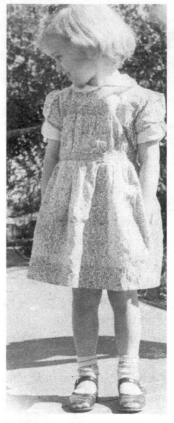

At age three, imagining my life's adventures, 1950

we were toddlers, was inspirational and big-hearted as well as a very humble and spiritual person. He showered his granddaughters with love and laughter, told us adventure stories that remained vivid in our imaginations, and played endless games with us. Ga-um even built a nine-hole miniature golf course around our rustic summer cabin in the Santa Cruz Mountains. As we worked on mastering the game, the giant redwood trees in the middle of the course provided additional challenges. Meanwhile, "Grammie" made sure that we had plenty of cookies, cakes, and pies to eat. This was undoubtedly the origin of my "sweet tooth."

Another precious gift from Ga-um were the letters and poems he wrote to my sister and me on our birthdays and during the periods we were apart, complete with illustrations. These are treasures that I enjoy reading once a year. After doting on his granddaughters, Ga-um enthusiastically welcomed a grandson and another Henry Shires into the family less than a year before he died.

My father, Henry M. Shires, was the only child of Ga-um and Grammie. He, too, was a remarkable man—brilliant, kind and compassionate, a gifted teacher and writer, and a wonderful father and pastor. His broad, warm smile was one of his trademarks. He was also extremely well organized and efficient. In contrast to our grandparents who spoiled us, our father was there to take disciplinary action when needed. We all looked up to him and tried to follow his wise counsel. I, along with my sister and brother, learned many important life lessons from him.

When he was 13, my father came down with polio but unlike his friends who faced the same terrible disease, he survived miraculously without paralysis as a result of an experimental treatment. He graduated early from high school and took advantage of the extra time before college to study jazz, expanding his love of music. Playing the piano, both classical and jazz, was one of my father's lifelong passions, especially when he needed a break from work. My father ended up majoring in French at Stanford University and then followed a similar career path as his father. He obtained a Master of Divinity, was an ordained minister in the Episcopal Church, and a few years later earned a Doctorate of Theology.

While he was Rector of three Episcopal parishes early in his career, my father was primarily an academic, teaching at the former Episcopal Theological School in Cambridge, Massachusetts for 22 years. During this period, he wrote several scholarly books on the New Testament. He also looked forward to his pastoral work each weekend. On Saturdays, he would write his sermon for the next day while watching college football or another favorite sport on TV. I marveled at how he managed to do both at the same time.

My mother's side of the family was notable for its spirited and fearless women. My maternal grandmother (Elizabeth Judkins) was an indomitable individual. Beginning in the 1920s, she successfully juggled, on her own, a career and two kids with little money and help. Loie (my mother) and her brother, Tod, were ages five and three when their parents divorced. At that time, divorce was highly stigmatized. Not only was it difficult for my grandmother but also for my mother and uncle who only saw their father occasionally.

I was named after my maternal grandmother who was known by her friends and colleagues as Liz. My independent streak came from "Grammie J" (as we called her), who passed this trait on to my mother and siblings along with her strong determination and boundless energy. Growing up, I was fortunate to spend time each summer with Ga-um and both grandmothers as well as with other family members in California.

I only remember seeing my maternal grandfather a few times before he died, including during a memorable visit to Washington, D.C. when I was a young girl to visit the major landmarks. My grandfather, who was a lawyer, worked for the U.S. Government as Chief of the International Trade Division in the Department of Commerce. All four grandparents had the opportunity to travel extensively overseas, which undoubtedly had an influence on my future career choice.

My mother was vivacious, warm, and generous. At 5'2", she was a foot shorter than my father and nine years younger; she brought complementary skills to the marriage and an outgoing personality. She was a superb hostess of events for parishioners, students, and faculty. My mother also spent a great deal of time during her life volunteering for social causes. If she had been born at another time and under different circumstances, she would have loved having a career. Like my grandparents and father, my mother always looked forward to travelling and occasionally took international trips on her own to visit friends. My mother and I were kindred spirits in terms of height and personality. We had a close and affectionate relationship, especially during my adulthood up until the time she died at age 90.

I am fortunate to have two wonderful siblings—Stephanie, who is three and a half years older, and Henry who is 13 years younger than I am. While my brother was a "surprise" for my parents, he was welcomed with great excitement into the family in 1960. My father was thrilled to have a son, and Stephanie and I were eager to have a brother. My mother reportedly asked the doctor right after the delivery, "What is she?" The doctor responded, "She's a he." My mother was apparently in a state of shock initially, commenting that she only knew how to take care of girls. However, she was delighted to have another Henry in the family and happy to have three children and later three grandchildren plus five great-grandchildren.

My family lived in Cambridge, Massachusetts (except for a few sabbaticals) for nine months of the year from the time I was in the third grade through my college years and beyond. When we travelled to California for summer vacations, we packed the car and headed west the day after school ended. Our collie occupied most of the back seat, leaving little room for the kids. Three months later, we returned to Cambridge just before classes resumed. My father always followed the same route across the country and kept to a strict schedule. The trip took us five days, with no time to visit interesting landmarks along the way.

In 1976, my parents moved back to California where my father returned to pastoral work before he died suddenly of a heart attack at the age of 67. We were devastated to lose him and the opportunity to share more of our adult years with him. His death was especially hard on my brother who was only 20 years old at the time.

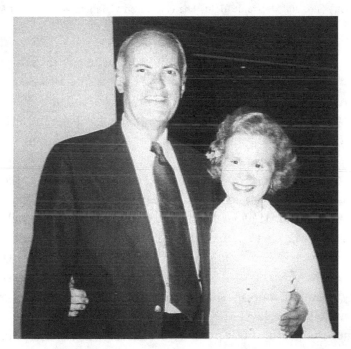

Dad and Mom, mid-1970s

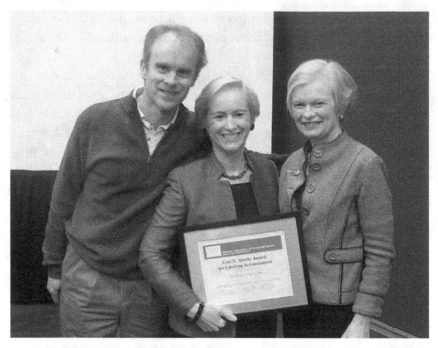

With Henry (left) and Stephanie (right) when I received a Lifetime Achievement Award from the American Public Health Association, 2013

Stephanie, Henry, and I look as though we belong to the same family and have certain distinct characteristics of our parents. However, each of us is unique. We have remained close over the years but have followed our own paths in life. Stephanie was a Classics major in college and an English teacher in addition to being a great mother and grandmother.

I was fascinated by romance languages and determined to pursue an international career. Henry took a different route as well, excelling in math and science. He majored in college in physics and has had a lifelong love of hiking, which included walking the entire Pacific Crest Trail (2,650 miles), from Mexico to Canada, as well as trekking in the Himalayas and Europe, among other places. Following his passion and using his many talents, Henry created his own company Tarptent, Inc., which makes high-quality, ultralight tents for serious hikers and all who want to maximize their outdoor experience.

Since the death of our parents, the three of us have kept in close touch—talking on the phone or via Skype and getting together whenever possible—although we live 700 and 3,000 miles apart. We enjoy reminiscing about our childhood, our parents and grandparents, and our different lives yet common bonds. I love being the aunt of a niece, Liz, and two nephews, Chris and Stuart, along with four great-nephews (Clark, Ben, Lucas, and Graham) and one great-niece (Maddie). They are all talented and lots of fun.

2

Pivotal Moments
in My Youth

Although we did not have much extra money growing up, our parents placed a premium on education and broadening our horizons. They were supportive of each of us pursuing our own interests, which for me, beginning at a young age, included travelling abroad and learning French. My first opportunity to go overseas happened when I was only four years old and we moved to England for the academic year, 1951–1952. My father was a postdoctoral researcher at the University of Oxford.

This was the first defining moment in my life. Stephanie and I had the exciting experience of living in another country, appreciating a different culture, going to a local school, and enjoying new friends and adventures. The British accents we picked up were later recorded by Grammie J. and were the source of much laughter in later years. During our time in England, we lived on food rations in a house with little heat and saw bomb-shattered London and other cities six years after the end of World War II. Along with meat once a week, our daily food staples were cauliflower, Brussels sprouts, and cabbage. As a small child, I hated these vegetables and have avoided eating them ever since.

From our base in Oxford, we toured other parts of England and Wales. We also travelled to France to visit our French cousins. The connection is a distant one via marriage. My great-aunt's sister-in-law (Elizabeth Witter) married a Frenchman, Henri Debost, following World War I when she was serving in the Red Cross and he was in the French military. In World War II, they escaped from Paris with three of their four young children to their summer home in the tiny village of Trouhaut, 17 miles northwest of Dijon in Burgundy. While they were in Trouhaut, their house was occupied by German soldiers. My relatives had to feed and cater to the soldiers' needs, although there was little to eat, and basic provisions were in scarce supply. The family's oldest son was in California right before the war began and ended up living with his American cousins for the duration of the war, including spending time with my mother.

Since my mother wanted us to meet the Debost family, she and a friend drove Stephanie and me to Burgundy while my father stayed behind in Oxford. Although I was very young, I have recollections of an adventurous trip from England to France, including a rough ferry ride and witnessing

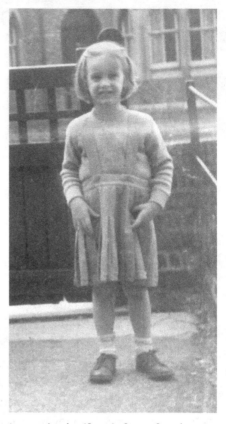

In my school uniform in front of our house in Oxford, 1952

the destruction of World War II along the way. Once in Trouhaut, we stayed at the Debost manor house, which dominated the tiny village.

The visit left a big impression on me at age five. I remember drinking milk from the family's cows and eating cheese for the first time as well as enjoying listening to a foreign language where I only knew a few basic expressions. I made friends with a local farm girl. Somehow, we managed to communicate and play together although we didn't speak each other's language. My time there sparked a strong interest in learning French, which became an enduring passion. I was fortunate to have the opportunity to study French in school beginning in the fifth grade and was inspired by a dynamic young teacher from Paris. I had other excellent French professors during my youth.

Another pivotal moment occurred when I turned 13. Grammie J. gave me a voluminous book on Africa for my birthday, which left an indelible mark. I became engrossed in reading about the history and culture of each country and marveled at the photos of this large, diverse, and fascinating continent where some countries were beginning to emerge from the yoke of colonialism. I decided at that point what I really wanted to do with my life: to travel and work internationally. Of course, at age 13, I had no idea what path this dream would take.

I sought more opportunities to travel during my teenage years when my family lived in Oxford again when I was 15. During that period, I spent more time in France and somehow talked my parents into letting me visit Paris for a week on my own, staying in my cousins' apartment although they were away. I toured Paris during the day and had dinner every evening with the concierge of the apartment building. My parents looked back at that time and wondered how they could have allowed me to tour the "City of Light" by myself as a young teenager. On each subsequent trip to France, visiting my cousins was a high priority. I loved seeing them and was always moved by their stories about what they experienced during World War II.

During the summer of my junior year in high school, I studied French for a month in Vichy, a famous spa town and seat of the Pétain government during World War II. When I was there, however, I did not know many of the details yet of the atrocities that had taken place throughout Europe only two decades earlier and the infamous reputation of Vichy. At the completion of my program, I received a "Certificat de Hautes Études" from the Centre International de Vichy, affiliated with the University of Clermont-Ferrand.

Before leaving Vichy, I was asked to be the guest speaker at a luncheon at the local Lions Club. However, when the time arrived for me to give my speech in French, I had come down with a bad case of laryngitis. Although they could barely hear me, the members of the Vichy Lions Club were understanding and gracious hosts. They gave me a cookbook, *La Cuisine du Monde*, which I still have 56 years later. Unfortunately, despite all the time in France and many other countries, cooking has never been one of my great interests or talents even though I have always appreciated cuisines from around the world.

When it was time to apply to college, I decided that I wanted to attend a small co-ed college in the northeast, having spent 11 years studying at a small private girls' school. Somehow, I ended up selecting Hobart and William Smith College in Geneva, New York over Middlebury College, which was also at the top of my list. My decision was heavily influenced by what I perceived to be a better social environment and the fact that Stephanie and her husband lived in the area rather than the result of a careful reflection about which college would be better for an aspiring French major. Luckily, I had some wonderful French professors at William Smith along with other excellent teachers. I also developed lifelong friendships with Lindley, Bonnie, and Judith, among others, and ended up in a serious relationship with Mike, the captain of the football and lacrosse teams.

At the end of my sophomore year in college, I spent another captivating summer abroad, this time travelling throughout Western Europe with my roommate, Lindley. We had a series of adventures during our whirlwind trip and struggled to stay within our budgetary limit of $10 a day. Some of the most memorable moments were visiting my cousins in Burgundy, seeing my parents and young brother in Florence (where my father was completing a sabbatical), and touring East Berlin, which felt eerily deserted and alien. In 1967, East Berlin was still behind the "Iron Curtain," and we were only allowed to be there for about five hours. We spent most of the time visiting the magnificent Pergamon Museum with its amazing antiquities collection. After our visit, we were very hungry and wandered the silent streets, in vain, trying to find a restaurant. On the bus back, we were once again thoroughly searched at the border crossing and were relieved to be back in vibrant West Berlin.

Early that fall, I began to make plans to study abroad again—for the second half of my junior year. I missed being in or near a large cosmopolitan area and wanted to learn another language and experience life in a country other than the U.K. and France. In the mid-1960s, study abroad programs were a new phenomenon. However, I was determined to take part in this experiment. After researching my options, I applied to a program in Florence run by Syracuse University because it was the only one that gave each student the opportunity to live with an Italian family rather than in a dorm with other Americans.

I made plans for my next overseas adventure without first consulting my parents or the Head of the French Department at Hobart and William Smith, fearing that my idea would be rejected. When I was accepted into the program, I was relieved when my French professor graciously granted me an exception to spend the rest of the academic year studying Italian, provided I submit a long paper in French before leaving. My parents were supportive of my plans as well, having been assured that there would be no increase in tuition.

One's destination is never a place, but a new way of seeing things.
—HENRY MILLER

The experience in Florence turned out to be a fantastic opportunity for personal growth and adventure. I woke up every morning saying "Buongiorno, Firenze" and embraced each day with excitement. During the week, I attended all my morning and late afternoon classes. The rest of the time I saw as much of the city as I could on foot and by bus—absorbing the language, culture, art, food, and sights.

I stayed with two quite different Italian families during that five-month period. My first family welcomed me like the daughter they never

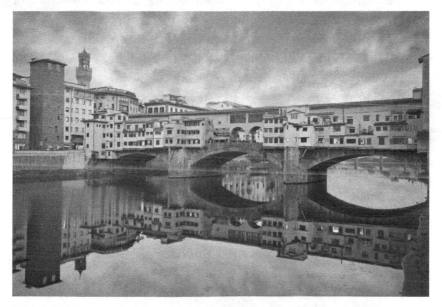

Part of my daily routine, gazing at the Ponte Vecchio. ISTOCK.COM / XAVIERAMAU

had. The couple was extremely kind and took good care of me. However, I was struck by the disparities in their roles. "La mia mamma" labored all day without a break—shopping, cooking, and cleaning. My "papà" had a completely different routine. After a light breakfast, he left each morning to meet with friends at a local café before going to work, returning home around 1pm for a delicious and copious lunch, which I enjoyed as well. Following a long siesta, he went back to his office around 4:30pm and then spent more time in the café on his way home. After a late supper, my papà would read the newspaper, smoke a cigar, and head to bed, while my mamma spent several more hours in the kitchen cleaning up and preparing for the next day.

When I joined the family, my papà stated that his goal was to turn me into a real Italian woman, noting that I was too thin and lacked the appropriate curves. He made sure that I ate heartily at every meal. Despite consuming more food than I had ever done before, along with ice cream between meals, I didn't gain any weight, much to his chagrin. While there, I also had my first introduction to the importance of calcio (soccer) in Italy and throughout Europe. The main soccer stadium in Firenze was only a block from the apartment. When there was an important match in the evening, it was hard to get to sleep because of all the celebrating or mourning in the streets, depending on the final score.

My second family lived on the top floor of an old apartment building located in the center of the city, a block from the famous Duomo. The head of the household was a hard-working widow in her late 40s who managed to care, on her own, for 18-year-old girl triplets plus a son in his early twenties studying at the local university. Her responsibilities expanded when a Swiss exchange student and I joined the family. The conversations around the large table in the kitchen were always lively and the food abundant. The meals included such foreign items to me as mozzarella, octopus, calamari, tripe (the edible lining of a cow's stomach), truffles, and roasted uccelli (baby birds) plus a large variety of pasta, bread, and soup that I had never tasted before. The seven of us shared a relatively small apartment and one bathroom. I often had to go to school early just to be able to wash up.

Meanwhile, back in the U.S., my parents complained that they had not received many letters from me, and that it was too expensive to talk on the phone. They were right. I hadn't kept in touch with them as frequently as I should have because of my full agenda. I had little free time between the hours I spent on my studies and sightseeing, as well as with my boyfriend, Guglielmo. From that point on, I started to write letters to my parents in Italian, which they both understood, to demonstrate that I was studying hard. My mother kept these letters for over four decades until we found them after she died.

On most weekends, I headed out of Firenze with friends, hitchhiking to other parts of the country, something which my parents would not likely have approved. I managed to see a great deal of Italy and experienced many adventures. My wanderlust was well nourished during that period. I also ended up speaking Italian quite well, including conversing using only hand gestures. Unfortunately, since my time in Italy, I have never been able to break the habit of speaking without using my hands a lot. This has, undoubtedly, been puzzling, if not disconcerting, to many people.

It was the first half of 1968 when I studied in Florence with strikes and protests throughout Italy. Similar events were occurring in other European countries I visited on my way home. When I returned to the U.S., it was not only the height of Vietnam War protests but also a momentous period for the civil rights movement. I was away during the terrible trauma that followed the assassinations of Dr. Martin Luther King, Jr. and Bobby Kennedy.

Back on campus in the fall of 1968, I felt as though I had missed a pivotal moment in U.S. history. Along with many others on campus, I joined in regular anti-war demonstrations. It was important to exercise our right to freedom of speech and assembly. We were all deeply concerned about whether our male classmates would be drafted and forced to participate in a war they did not support. Some of our friends were willing to serve. Others lived in fear of receiving a low draft number and anguished over whether they should become conscientious objectors and move to Canada.

Despite the turmoil on campus, my senior year went by quickly. In addition to completing my courses as a French major, I taught French for a semester at a local high school and obtained my teaching certificate. My classes ranged from introductory to advanced French. I had students who hated having to learn a foreign language, including most members of the football team. Rather than focusing on the course material I had prepared, they ended up sitting in the front row and staring at my miniskirts. Fortunately, there were other students who loved French and engaged in the classes enthusiastically. Trying to meet the needs and interests of a wide range of students tested my ingenuity and was another opportunity for personal growth.

At graduation, after all my partying—particularly during my freshman and sophomore years—and the money spent on my college education, my father expressed his appreciation that it had been worth it when I was inducted into the local chapter of Phi Beta Kappa. This honor meant a lot to him since he was proud to have received it decades earlier at Stanford University.

3

OPENING A NEW CHAPTER
AND FINDING MY PARTNER

My main goal in 1969 was to launch the "international career" I had dreamed about since the age of 13. After graduation, I went on another trip to France to see my cousins in Burgundy and some other parts of the country I had not visited before. Then, in mid-summer, I packed up and moved to Washington, D.C. This was only the second time in my life that I had travelled to the nation's capital. I had to find a place to stay, a roommate to share the rent, and, most importantly, a job. Since 1969 was well before personal computers and the internet, I undertook a thorough search in the D.C. phonebook of all the international organizations in the area. I then visited the ones I found most interesting.

I was excited to receive an offer from Voice of America, part of the U.S. Information Agency. The position was Assistant to the Chief of the French Branch of the Africa Division—combining my two great interests at the time. However, before starting work, I had to pass a typing test, which was mandatory for all women even though the job for which I applied was not a secretarial one. I had never taken a typing class in high school and had to teach myself. Although my typing was not great, I managed to pass the test by one point.

I learned a lot in a very stimulating, fast-paced work environment where I was the only American and one of only two women in a newsroom of male French and African journalists. I provided a range of services in support of the daily four and a half hours of French-language radio broadcasts for Francophone sub-Saharan Africa. Part of my job was to identify and review source materials, respond in French to questions from listeners, and analyze audience feedback. I was fascinated to learn that many listeners expressed great concern over the U.S. landing on the Moon in July 1969, believing that this historic event was going to upset the Universe and unleash evil spirits. My other responsibilities included providing French-English translations, as needed, serving as a periodic broadcaster on the daily program "Bonjour l'Afrique," assisting the radio producer, and helping conduct interviews of African dignitaries.

I also had a chance to interact with journalists who were broadcasting in Swahili as well as others involved in daily broadcasts in 36 different languages. I felt as though I was working in the United Nations and that I had landed my dream job, including being able to speak French every day.

While at VOA, I had another defining moment in my life: finding my husband and lifelong partner, Terry Maguire. We met in the fall of 1969 through one of my roommates whose cousin was enrolled in the U.S. Coast Guard Officer Candidate School (OCS) along with Terry. Rebounding from my first great love in college and not interested in the current guy I was dating (except his sports car), I was attracted especially by Terry's intellect as well as his interest in becoming an international media lawyer. My mother thought he looked like Robert Redford. After graduating from OCS, Terry was given the choice of working at U.S. Coast Guard headquarters in Washington, D.C. or commanding a patrol boat on the Mekong Delta in Vietnam. In a heartbeat, he picked the first option and moved to the nation's capital a few months after we met.

The next year we spent a lot of time together in between our work obligations. Terry was writing speeches for the Commandant of the U.S. Coast Guard and working on Coast Guard regulations during the day. In the evenings he was enrolled in a master's degree program in Communications at American University. We were married in December 1970 in Cambridge, Massachusetts, with my father presiding over the ceremony. Afterwards, Terry also completed his law studies at night at George Washington University, passed the bar exam in D.C. and Florida, and then specialized in media law.

Terry and I had complementary personalities and were pursuing different careers. However, we shared common political philosophies, a zest for learning, and a passion for international work and travelling. This bond has remained solid over a life full of adventures, opportunities, and some challenges.

In counselling us before we were married, my father underscored the importance of continuing to grow each year as individuals as well as building our relationship as a couple. We have tried to follow his wise advice over the past five decades.

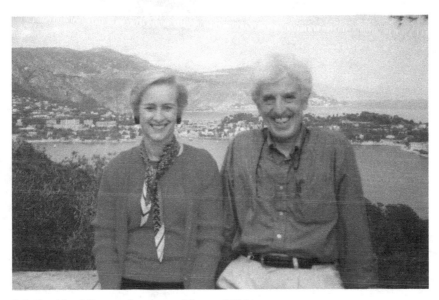

Enjoying Nice 30 years after our wedding, c. 2000

PART TWO

Pursuing a Global Mission

INCREASING ACCESS TO FAMILY PLANNING
AND REPRODUCTIVE HEALTH

4

POPULATION REFERENCE BUREAU (PRB)

In following my passions, I was able to find my mission in life—through perseverance and serendipity.

While I was happy at Voice of America, I decided that I did not want to be a journalist or radio broadcaster. I was still searching for a career with a meaningful global mission. After two years at VOA, a friend asked if I would be interested in a position at the Population Reference Bureau (PRB) based in Washington, D.C. PRB was dedicated to educating audiences in the U.S. and overseas about population trends and related health issues, including family planning. In the fall of 1971, the organization was looking for someone with experience in Francophone Africa to help launch and oversee a publications program in French for the region, similar to the Spanish and Portuguese publications for Latin American audiences. Based on my knowledge of French-speaking Africa, proficiency in French, and a strong interest in PRB's work, I was offered the job.

As soon as I arrived at PRB in November 1971, I was asked to undertake a feasibility study of whether there was enough interest in Francophone West Africa for publications in French on population, health, and family planning issues. I began compiling a list, in consultation with others, of key people to interview and was ready to leave on my first trip to Africa in 1972. The itinerary included stops in Senegal, Mali, Côte d'Ivoire, Ghana, Togo, and Benin. I was glad that Terry was able to accompany me on this big adventure.

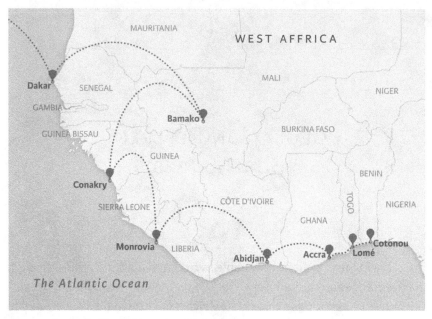

Our travel route in West Africa, 1972. DNC Maps

We took a non-stop flight from New York to Dakar, Senegal and were among the few non-Africans on board. In Dakar, my round of visits included talking to health care officials, educators, and journalists. One of the memorable meetings was with staff of the only family planning clinic in sub-Saharan Francophone Africa, La Croix Bleue. This was my first introduction to the importance of offering women family planning information and services so that they could plan the number and spacing of their children and achieve other goals in life. And yet, the number of women this one clinic could serve was miniscule in comparison to the demand.

I also visited the main teaching hospital in Dakar, which was overcrowded and poorly equipped. The staff were clearly unable to attend to all the people inside the hospital facilities, let alone all those lying outside. As I mentioned in the Introduction, it was on the grounds of this hospital where I witnessed a young woman hemorrhaging from an unsafe abortion. The death of this powerless Senegalese woman was another defining moment in my life. It inspired me to seek opportunities where I could help other women avoid a similar fate. As I began to study this issue, I learned that enabling women to prevent and manage safely unwanted pregnancies was an area of huge unmet need throughout the world.

I became a passionate advocate for the right of every woman to control her fertility at a time when these issues were being hotly debated in the U.S. leading up to the 1973 Supreme Court decision on Roe v. Wade. As we continued our journey in West Africa, I was anxious to learn more about maternal deaths and injuries due to unsafe abortion and the importance of providing a range of contraceptive choices for women.

Along with the many interesting meetings we had, Terry and I were fascinated by the rich culture and customs, historical sites, markets, crafts, and cuisine of each country. We also had many adventures along the way. Our first night in Dakar, when we were adjusting to jet lag, we were awakened suddenly before sunrise with the call to prayer by a *muezzin*. We hadn't realized that our small hotel was next to a mosque.

After spending five days in Senegal, we took a late afternoon flight to Bamako, the capital of Mali. As we were nearing our destination on a clear night, we could not see any bright lights shining below, nor were there any lights on the runway as we touched down, other than some large candles. The airport turned out to be a small building with a thatched roof. Our hotel, one of only a few in the capital, was a former brothel—and perhaps continues to be one. There were just six rooms upstairs with one bathroom at the end of the hall. The "Madame" was sitting at the bar, as she had likely been doing for many years when the hotel was frequented by members of the French Foreign Legion.

We loved touring the large market in the center of town, full of colorful beads and magnificent carvings. Later, we purchased a beautiful Dogon carving to remind us of our time in Mali.

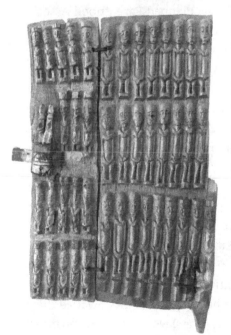

Dogon granary door with carved ancestral figures to ward off evil spirits

However, while in Bamako, we were almost arrested twice, once for taking a photo of a bridge that we didn't realize was forbidden. The second time we were given a warning for walking too close to the presidential palace. As we waited for our plane to take off from Bamako several days later, we noticed that the pilot had been drinking at the bar for well over an hour. When we were ready to board our flight, we watched him stumble up the stairway and into the cockpit. Terry and I were unsure whether we would ever make it to our next destination.

En route to Côte d'Ivoire, we had brief stops in Conakry, Guinea, and Monrovia, Liberia. When we finally landed safely in Abidjan, we were very relieved. Our time in the capital of Côte d'Ivoire passed quickly with a series of productive meetings and clinic visits related to my work assignment. The rest of the time we spent touring the capital, marveling at a few modern high-rise buildings next to sprawling slums.

Our next destination, Accra, Ghana, was quite different from the other capitals we visited. It was reminiscent of its former colonial power, Great Britain, with narrow streets and roundabouts. A highlight of our time was meeting with dedicated staff at the Ghana Planned Parenthood Association founded five years earlier by Professor Fred Sai, one of the world's great pioneers in championing women's reproductive health and rights.

After Accra, we drove to Lomé, Togo to meet with other officials and then on to Cotonou, the largest city and port in Benin. We knew we were back in former French colonies when we saw wide avenues and ate French-inspired cuisine. Outside the urban areas, however, we were struck by endless lines of women walking on the side of the road. Each one was carrying a large bucket of water or bundle of wood on her head, along with a baby on her back and often another one in her belly. While the women were working from dawn to dusk, we noticed the men either relaxing under a tree or spending time in a café. This picture is one that I saw many times in every country I visited throughout my career.

Another unforgettable and searing experience during our more than five-week trip to West Africa was visiting the forts in Ghana and Senegal where men and women were once held captive as they awaited their journeys across the Atlantic Ocean to serve as slaves in the U.S. and other destinations in the region. This was a sober reminder of one of the darkest chapters in the history of the U.S.

When I returned to PRB after my African travels and finished my report, I concluded that launching a French-language publications program on population and family planning issues was premature. The French anti-contraception law of 1920 was still in effect in Francophone Africa, and there was strong opposition to family planning among a wide range of stakeholders—except for some dedicated health care providers and women who desperately needed these life-saving and life-enhancing services. PRB was also unable to secure sufficient funding.

Because I was not going to be able to use my French as planned, I ended up studying Spanish in the evenings in order to work on PRB's program for Latin America. Learning Spanish and some Portuguese was easy for me after a background in French and Italian. As Director of Media Programs for Latin America, I launched a biweekly population news feature, *Qué Pasa*, for broadcast and print media. I had the chance to work with journalists in Central and South America who were interested in writing about population, health, and family planning issues. I subsequently helped write and edit a monthly newsletter, *Población*, for Latin American decision makers, which included a Portuguese version. I also developed materials for a bilingual monthly bulletin for English-language teachers in Brazil.

Through these initiatives, I had the opportunity to travel to several countries in the Western Hemisphere where I met some of the great family planning pioneers. It was a privilege to spend time with dynamic leaders from Colombia, notably Dr. Fernando Tamayo, who founded the family planning organization, Profamilia, and Dr. Jorge Villarreal, from the Colombian Association of Medical Schools (ASCOFAME) and subsequent founder of Oriéntame, offering comprehensive reproductive health services, including safe, legal abortion. I also met with Dr. Guillermo López Escobar, who was head of the Division of Population Studies at ASCOFAME.

In addition, I greatly admired Dr. Benjamin Viel, an eminent Chilean professor of public health and an outspoken champion of women's right to contraception. He played a pivotal role in training medical students and obstetricians-gynecologists (ob-gyns) in family planning. Another impressive leader was Dr. Roberto Santiso-Gálvez, one of the founding members of APROFAM, the private family planning association of Guatemala. In 1974, I witnessed the great excitement when Mexico made family planning a constitutional right of all couples.

In the early to mid-70s, family planning was highly controversial throughout the Latin American region due to the strong opposition from the Catholic hierarchy. The courageous leaders I met represented the first of a long list of brilliant, dedicated, and charismatic men and women who were sources of inspiration throughout my career in advancing women's reproductive health and rights.

One of the other passionate family planning leaders I encountered while I was at PRB was Dr. George Brown. At that time, he was working for the Canadian-sponsored International Development Research Centre. Our paths crossed many times during my career while he was serving as Vice President of International Programs at the Population Council in New York City for 24 years.

I found the work environment at PRB to be fun and stimulating, especially in the International Programs Department where I had young female colleagues from Puerto Rico and Chile as well as a Canadian, Roslyn Hees, who became a lifelong friend. Our boss, the Director of International Programs, was a talented journalist from Colombia with a volatile personality; he was very engaging and charming much of the time, but when his temper surfaced, it was not pleasant.

After working at PRB for a couple of years, I decided, along with a few other brave employees, to seek a private meeting with the Chair of the Board. We were concerned about what seemed to be possible financial irregularities by our boss, although we had little data. Once we had the appointment, we took great care to sneak out of the office, knowing that we risked being fired. Fortunately, this did not happen, and the Board Chair listened intently to our concerns and the limited information available to us. He followed up immediately, and a few months later, the FBI showed up and escorted our boss out of the office. The valuable lesson for me, and my colleagues, was that it is important to speak up and take action when you sense something is wrong.

In September 1974, I was appointed Acting Director of International Programs, supervising a staff of 12. Having an expanded scope of work was exciting and rewarding. I directed activities of the Latin American Department, with overall responsibility for editing five Spanish-language publications (circulation 20,000) for a Latin American audience. These publications covered a wide range of topics featuring new developments in population, family planning, and related fields.

By the spring of 1975, I decided that it was time for graduate school, and I enrolled in the master's degree program in demography and sociology at Georgetown University. I left PRB in June of that year to begin my studies, not knowing that 30 years later, I would serve on the Board of Trustees of this wonderful organization.

5

GEORGETOWN UNIVERSITY

In the summer of 1975, I was eager to begin my first graduate course. Although I had been a liberal arts undergraduate major, I was looking forward to stretching my mind and taking biostatistics and demography, including courses on fertility and mortality, among others. I was pleased that my first course was on international family planning programs. I found it fascinating.

In mid-July, Terry and I took a break one weekend and visited his family on Long Island. Taking advantage of the lovely weather, we went on a 25-mile bike ride and had a great time. When we returned to D.C., I began experiencing pain in my lower back and left leg. I thought that I was just out of shape. However, over the next week, I became progressively worse and had some difficulty walking. My doctor felt that I might have something more serious than just strained muscles.

Since this was before the invention of magnetic resonance imaging, I was admitted to a local hospital and scheduled for a myelogram. The procedure involved injecting dye into my spinal canal and taking x-rays. I remember the neurosurgeon commenting with alarm that I had a large tumor on my spinal cord — something extremely rare that he had only seen once before. He thought it had been growing for over 10 years. This was likely the source of my periodic back pain in high school and college. I was active in several team sports and always dismissed the discomfort.

A lumbar laminectomy was scheduled immediately. I wanted to make sure, however, that I first took the final exam for my summer course. I managed to complete it in my hospital bed before the surgery. The operation was a very risky one, involving scraping the tumor off my spinal cord without damaging it. My family was told beforehand that I had a 50% chance of walking again.

I managed to beat the odds and came through the delicate procedure able to move my legs! The only complication I suffered was a slight weakness in my left leg and subsequent lower back pain and sciatica. Moreover, I was counselled that carrying a pregnancy could be difficult and was therefore not advisable. At that point, having children was not a high priority for us since we were both focused on our careers.

As I was regaining my strength from the surgery, I reflected on how fortunate I was to have access to expert surgeons and high-quality medical care when so much of the world's population does not enjoy the same right. I also developed great empathy for people who are not able to walk or use their legs without difficulty, for whatever reason. I could easily have found myself in the same situation. Throughout my time in the hospital and during my recovery at home, Terry was at my side. I was extremely grateful for his devoted care.

My health issues did not stop me from pursuing my passions in life. I was determined to resume my master's degree program when courses started again in September. Despite the surgery, I did not miss any of my classes and kept to my original timetable.

Although I thoroughly enjoyed my graduate work and learned a lot, I realized that I did not want to be a demographer in the U.S. Bureau of the Census or have a career in academia. My most interesting course was the one on family planning taught by Dr. Joe Speidel. At the time, he was serving as Director of the Research Division in the Office of Population (now the Office of Population and Reproductive Health) at the U.S. Agency for International Development (USAID).

While I was pursuing my master's degree, Joe Speidel continued to urge me to join USAID. I finally relented a year later. I stipulated that I only wanted to work for the U.S. government for two years, preferring the more flexible, less bureaucratic environment of a non-profit organization. I ended up staying at USAID for the two years I promised plus 20 more. During that period, I had many opportunities to expand my knowledge, skills, and experience. Most importantly, I was able to contribute to a noble mission.

6

U.S. Agency for International Development (USAID)

In January 1977, I became a Population Research Scientist in the Research Division of the Office of Population. I was excited to start my new career in international family planning and reproductive health.

On my first day at USAID after I was sworn in as a government employee, I learned that I no longer had the boss who hired me. Joe Speidel had just been promoted to Associate Director of the Office. My new boss was Duff Gillespie, who did not know me and wasn't sure initially what role I would play in the Division. It was clear when I joined the Office of Population that I had to adjust once again to a heavily male-dominated environment where all those in positions of power were men. I was one of only a handful of professional women; the rest held secretarial positions.

My closest female colleagues during my first few years in the Office included Miriam Labbok, Barbara Kennedy, Sarah Clark, and Sara Seims—all extremely talented people who went on to have impressive careers. As women, we had to work even harder than our male colleagues to prove that we were just us as smart and effective—if not more so. We had to speak up—and sometimes act out—to be heard and become more valued. While it took years for real change to occur in terms of gender equity in the workplace, I nevertheless learned a lot from Duff and my other male bosses as well as from my female colleagues.

Soon after I joined, Duff asked me whether I spoke French and, if so, whether I wanted to attend a conference in Tunisia. I responded with an enthusiastic "oui." The international conference was the first of its kind on Household Distribution of Contraceptives, an initiative to take family planning information and services out of the clinic and make them more accessible to women. The conference in March 1977 greatly enhanced my knowledge of family planning and innovative ways of expanding the availability of this essential preventive care. It also provided an opportunity for me to interact with family planning leaders from around the world.

While in Tunis, I met the Minister of Public Health and key staff in charge of the national family planning program. I visited several US-AID-funded family planning service delivery sites in central Tunisia where I was able to witness first-hand the effectiveness of reaching women in their communities. After first gaining the consent of village chiefs, family planning officials trained young local women to serve as community outreach workers. Their job was to visit each household or compound to interview reproductive-age women, talk about contraception, offer birth control pills and condoms, keep records, and provide follow-up. As we accompanied several community workers on their rounds, I could see the level of interest expressed by almost every woman we visited and the sense of empowerment that came with having some control over her reproductive life despite initial resistance, in some cases, from her husband or mother-in-law.

The outreach workers played a critical role in supporting women in their communities and even accompanied them to the nearest clinic or hospital when needed. During my career, I visited countless community workers as well as health facilities and personnel throughout the developing world and always enjoyed these experiences.

My first trip to Tunisia in 1977 was the beginning of more than a decade-long working relationship with colleagues in the office overseeing the national family planning program, known as the Office National de la Famille et de la Population (ONFP). During this period, I interacted with health care personnel in Tunis and around the country. I was later appointed the focal point in USAID/Washington for the Agency's bilateral population assistance program to Tunisia aimed at improving the availability and quality of family planning services. I was grateful for the chance to spend a lot of time in this fascinating country and appreciate its rich culture and history. I developed wonderful friendships with Anwar Bachbaouab, Mohamed Ayad, Mongi Bchir, Fethi Ben Messaoud, Mourad Ghachem, and Hafedh Chekir, among others. Each trip offered new adventures and opportunities to learn and contribute. Moreover, I was able to use my French and learn some Arabic as well.

MEMORABLE EXPERIENCES

One of my most memorable experiences in Tunisia was an invitation to lunch in the early 1980s with President Habib Bourguiba and Prime Minister Mzali at the presidential palace. I had the great honor of being seated to the left of President Bourguiba and across from the prime minister. Our first course was a Tunisian specialty, *brik à l'oeuf*, which is a light pastry filled with an egg, capers, and herbs and cooked in hot oil until brown. I tried to eat it carefully so that none of the egg slipped through the pastry shell onto the plate. This would have been an embarrassing faux pas, especially in such a formal setting.

As we ate, President Bourguiba recounted the story of his mother who had delivered eight sons. He talked passionately about how much she had suffered through so many pregnancies. After becoming the country's first president following independence, Habib Bourguiba took the courageous move of granting women equal rights in 1956 with the passage of the Personal Status Code. The national family planning program was launched in mid-1966, following a two-year pilot initiative. Abortion in the first trimester was legalized in 1973. As a result of President Bourguiba's progressive actions, Tunisia was far ahead of other countries in the region, as well as most nations in the world, in advancing women's reproductive health and rights.

When I co-authored an article entitled "The Delivery and Use of Contraceptive Services in Rural Tunisia," published in *International Family Planning Perspectives* in September 1982, I noted that abortion was legal in Tunisia. However, because I had mentioned the word "abortion," a sensitive topic during the Reagan Administration, I was subsequently investigated by a senior USAID political appointee. My files on Tunisia were confiscated, and I received a reprimand in my personnel file. This was a shocking development since I had only mentioned a simple fact in writing about Tunisia. What happened to "freedom of speech" and reporting the truth? The only silver lining was that the reprimand did not impede my career at USAID. In fact, it became my "badge of honor," which I noted in my remarks at my retirement party years later.

During my first eight years at USAID, I was primarily involved in the operations research program, aimed at increasing the accessibility and cost-effectiveness of family planning services. I was responsible for overseeing initially a $12 million, five-year technical assistance program administered by Columbia University, under the supervision of Dr. Allan Rosenfield, a world renowned ob-gyn, who was Director of the Center for Family Health and later Dean of the Mailman School of Public Health at Columbia University. He was a visionary with a great sense of humor.

I had an opportunity to work with Allan and especially with several of his staff on the design, implementation, and evaluation of innovative family planning and maternal and child health service delivery systems in Africa, the Near East, Latin America, and the Caribbean. Some of my earliest visits were to Haiti, where the needs were overwhelming. I was impressed with the commitment of local health care providers to save and improve the lives of women and children living in extreme poverty and challenging conditions.

In 1980, I travelled to Zaire (now the Democratic Republic of the Congo, or DRC), a country covering an area of over 905,000 square miles, the largest in sub-Saharan Africa. The purpose of my trip was to work with a young professor from Tulane University, Dr. Jane Bertrand, who was the principal investigator on another USAID-funded operations research project. While Jane and I had talked on the phone, we only really got to know each other when we arrived in Zaire and were getting ready to travel from Kinshasa to the remote village of Nsona Mpangu in the southwestern tip of the country. Jane's husband, Bill, negotiated with a driver to take Jane and me on the long ride to our destination. To pay for the transport, we had to turn over the contents of a small suitcase of local bills, given the hyperinflation at the time.

Before we got underway, the driver had to buy extra gas to last the entire journey. He put it in a topless large steel drum behind the back seat of the station wagon and immediately lit a cigarette. In fact, he smoked continuously during the day-long trip, while the gas was sloshing around in the open barrel directly behind our heads. Despite our objections, the driver made it clear that if we wanted him to do his job, he was going to keep smoking, as it calmed his nerves. It is amazing that we survived the journey without being blown up!

This was my first time in rural Zaire. As we neared our destination, we saw a group of young boys surrounding our car shouting "Mundele!" or "white people!" We were, indeed, a rare sight in that area. While we were in the small community of Nsona Mpangu, we stayed in a simple brick dwelling. At night, I found it hard to get to sleep and was reluctant to get out of my cot because there were bats circling overhead and rats scurrying around on the floor. Jane, who had stayed there on previous trips, was not bothered by this at all. Apart from the plentiful mangoes from the trees around us, our food options were limited, and I often felt hungry. One evening we were treated to a specialty of the region – *chimérique*. It turned out to be a large river rat, which was roasted with its full head of hair. I could barely look at it, let alone eat it! It was impossible to consume more than a few bites without gagging while trying to be respectful to our hosts.

During our time in the bush, we met with community leaders and health care workers in the surrounding villages. The operations research project seemed to be well accepted and effective in terms of increasing awareness and acceptance of family planning and maternal-child health care.

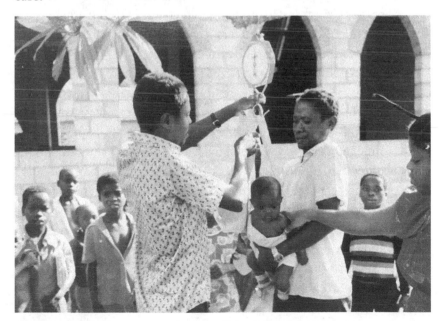

A health worker in the Nsona Mpangu area, Zaire, 1980s. JANE BERTRAND

On one of our daily outings, we saw a very distraught couple whose young son had just fallen out of a mango tree and was severely injured from a root that had pierced his abdomen. Since we had a truck, we all drove immediately back to the small field hospital in Nsona Mpangu to see if the doctor could save the boy's life.

Due to the seriousness of his injury and the lack of adequate equipment, the boy died on the operating table. We then witnessed the parents' enormous pain and grief. They attributed their son's death to the belief that someone in their village had cast an evil spell on them. We watched as they headed home to determine who should pay for the tragic loss of their son. The death of loved ones who are unable to receive adequate medical care is sadly a common occurrence for families throughout the developing world.

On the long trip back to Kinshasa, our truck was travelling on a winding road with a huge ravine on one side. Suddenly the driver hit the brakes. We looked up and saw an army tank with its long gun barrel pointed at us. We thought there had been a coup d'état while we were in Nsona Mpangu, where we did not have access to reliable communications. Instead, we quickly learned that the tank had broken down. Since the soldiers had not been paid in quite some time, they helped themselves to all the food and other items of interest in our truck, which was carrying other people back to Kinshasa. When the soldiers finally allowed us to continue our journey, we were able to breathe again!

On a lighter note, Jane and I realized at the beginning of our adventure that my husband, Terry, was the first person she dated as a freshman at Pembroke when he was a junior at Brown University. We shared many laughs over this coincidence as we became close friends, and we plotted how I would tell Terry when I returned to D.C. When I showed him the photos of my trip, I purposely put one of Jane on the top of the pile. I wish that I had captured on camera his stunned expression. Terry was aware that I was travelling with Jane Bertrand, but he only knew her by her maiden name (Trowbridge). He immediately searched among his old photos and showed me for the first time all the ones of the two of them together several years before we met and married.

In addition to extensive travel in Francophone Africa, I was able to spend more time in Latin America, which I had enjoyed immensely from my work at PRB. Early in my USAID career, I had the exciting experience of serving, on short-term basis, as Acting Population Officer at the U.S. Embassy in Mexico City. During this assignment, I met passionate health care providers and other leaders in Mexico, all committed to increasing women's access to quality family planning services.

While there, I visited one of the USAID-sponsored operations research projects in a large slum area on the outskirts of the capital, which served as the city's main dump. This district was home to more than one million people who worked from early morning to evening sifting through garbage and selling what they could salvage in an effort to survive from one day to the next. We supported the training of community outreach workers to provide information on family planning and other essential health services to this impoverished population; these workers served as a vital link to the nearest health clinic and often accompanied women and children to provide support. Witnessing this innovative initiative was another of a long list of memorable experiences.

One of the impressive leaders I met was Dr. Manuel Urbina who served at the time as head of the National Family Planning Coordinating Agency and later as secretary general of the Mexican National Population Council. Manuel and I have kept in touch over the past 40 years and served together on the Board of Pathfinder International.

Expanding Responsibilities

In early 1982, when I became Deputy Chief of the Research Division, my portfolio expanded to co-managing a staff of 14 and a $23 million worldwide population research program supporting contraceptive development and demographic research in addition to family planning operations research. Also, as the Director of Operations Research, I oversaw a major expansion of the program, which included 14 contracts with U.S. institutions and 53 projects in 26 developing countries.

The best part of the job continued to be the extensive travel and meeting remarkable people in every country. During almost all my travels, I spent time with women and their families in villages or slum areas of major cities along with dedicated health care providers and senior Ministry of Health officials. I wish that I had kept a written record of all these experiences, apart from the more technical trip reports I wrote.

Towards the end of 1984, I left the Research Division to become Chief of the Policy Development Division, where we supported demographic data collection and analysis, policy research, awareness-raising on population-development dynamics, and assistance to developing countries in the design and implementation of population policies. This was another opportunity for innovation and personal growth. I had a great staff when I arrived and was pleased that my old college friend and former PRB colleague, Judith Seltzer, became my deputy.

As a team, we addressed new program issues, reached new audiences, and experimented with new program approaches. One of the initiatives we launched was the IMPACT information and dissemination program, which ended up reaching decision makers in 100 countries. Another was a new policy initiative with the for-profit private sector. We also expanded population policy support to Africa. This assistance helped lead to policy changes in many countries in a three-year period. A particularly interesting experience was participating in a small private briefing in French for President Eyadéma of Togo, followed by a formal presentation to the National Assembly. Afterwards, I helped with the development of the country's first population policy, working with John May who has written extensively on population policies in Africa.

In February 1987, I attended the first International Safe Motherhood Conference in Nairobi, Kenya, a defining moment in addressing much-neglected maternal health problems in developing countries that also resulted in the launch of the Safe Motherhood Initiative. Dr. Allan Rosenfield co-authored a landmark paper on "Maternal mortality--a neglected tragedy: Where is the M in MCH?" At the conference, I not only saw my good friend Allan Rosenfield in action but was also inspired by the speeches of Professor Mahmoud Fathalla of Egypt as well as Professor Fred Sai of Ghana who served as moderator of the conference.

It is hard to imagine three more inspirational leaders—all pioneers in the field of women's reproductive health. Along with Dr. Rosenfield's distinguished service, Professor Fathalla was Dean of the Medical School of Assiut University in Egypt and held many senior positions during his career. He served as Director of the Special Programme of Research, Development and Research Training in Human Reproduction (HRP) at the World Health Organization (WHO); Senior Advisor for Biomedical and Reproductive Health and Research at the Rockefeller Foundation; and President of the International Federation of Gynecology and Obstetrics (FIGO), to mention just a few. Professor Fred Sai also held numerous key positions, including Professor of Preventive and Social Medicine at the University of Ghana Medical School, Director of the Ghana Health Service, President of the International Planned Parenthood Federation, and Senior Population Advisor at the World Bank. Towards the end of his career, Professor Sai advised the President of Ghana on reproductive health and HIV/AIDS. I was fortunate to have many more occasions to spend time with these charismatic leaders, as well as others, over the course of my career.

During my USAID years, I was given increasing opportunities for professional growth and leadership. At each stage, I helped other female colleagues advance as well. The work environment began to change as more women held positions of responsibility. In mid-1988, I became part of the executive management team of the Office of Population, serving first as Associate Director, and later in 1992, I was promoted to Deputy Director. Over these four years, I helped oversee the Office of Population's worldwide program and a budget increase of $100 million. I also managed much of the day-to-day operations of the Office of Population.

Other responsibilities involved guiding USAID-funded family planning activities in Latin America and the Caribbean, the Near East, and North Africa. I conducted strategic programming exercises in Mexico, Brazil, Morocco, and Tunisia with plans for gradual phase-out of financial support after many years of USAID assistance. I also opened a dialogue for the first time with the Algerian government on population and health issues.

While travelling, I continued to see important progress in many countries as a result of USAID family planning assistance. Throughout the developing world, the use of family planning increased, as did local government commitment to providing these vital services.

Another interesting aspect of my job was serving as a liaison to the UN Population Fund (UNFPA). I helped develop the Global Initiative on Contraceptive Requirements and Logistics Management Needs and represented USAID at the annual UNDP Governing Council reviews of UNFPA. This gave me a chance to spend time with Dr. Nafis Sadik, the dynamic Pakistani Executive Director of UNFPA, and her senior staff. Similar opportunities emerged to expand coordination with the World Bank, WHO, the International Planned Parenthood Federation, and other bilateral aid agencies.

From 1988–1992, I also served on the Board of Directors of the Sahel Institute's Center for Applied Research on Population and Development (CERPOD). I was the only woman and the only non-African working with directors and staff from the region. I was impressed by their dedication and skill, and by the warm welcome they gave me. It was a privilege to support the pioneering work of this organization and to attend Board meetings in different countries in the Sahel. The most fascinating venue for one of our meetings was Cape Verde, a former Portuguese colony and archipelago of 10 volcanic islands located 350 miles off the coast of Senegal in the Atlantic Ocean. In addition to enjoying meeting local dignitaries and the chance to speak Portuguese, I had the best lobster meal I have ever eaten.

BREAKING THE GLASS CEILING

In January 1993, I took over as head of the Office of Population at the beginning of the Clinton Administration. I was the first female director since the program started in the mid-1960s. I subsequently became a career member of the U.S. Government's Senior Executive Service.

In overseeing the world's largest international family planning assistance program during most of the 1990s, I felt privileged to work not only with a dedicated staff of 70 but also with a wide range of implementing agencies and many impressive Foreign Service officers and host country officials around the world. The Office of Population supported contraceptive research and development; contraceptive procurement and logistics management; family planning and reproductive health service delivery; management and training; communications; policy development; and data collection, research and evaluation. We managed a budget of over $250 million by the end of my tenure, representing 65% of USAID's population assistance, delivered through 46 multi-million-dollar agreements with U.S. institutions working in partnership with governments, non-governmental organizations, and commercial entities in over 60 developing countries.

THE INTERNATIONAL CONFERENCE ON POPULATION AND DEVELOPMENT (ICPD)

The most exciting period of my USAID career was participating in the landmark International Conference on Population and Development, held in Cairo, 5-13 September 1994.

I was active in preparatory events leading up to Cairo, including serving as Vice-Chair of the UN Expert Group Meeting on Family Planning, Health and Family Well-Being in Bangalore, India in October 1992. Participants included representatives from different geographic regions and scientific disciplines. Among the key topics addressed was the need to shift from demographic targets to the family planning and other reproductive health needs of individual women, along with attention to their status and the health and well-being of their families. The special needs of adolescents and the importance of greater male engagement in family planning were also highlighted. Public-private partnerships to meet contraceptive needs and increased resources were noted as priorities as well.

What made this experience especially rich was the opportunity to work closely with Professor Mahmoud Fathalla of Egypt, the "father of reproductive health," a brilliant and compassionate ob-gyn and eloquent speaker. As Chair of the Drafting Committee, I was extremely honored to have Professor Fathalla as a vital member of the group. His inspiration and wise counsel are reflected in all the recommendations for action, which provided a strong basis for key elements of the ICPD Programme of Action two years later. The biggest breakthrough was on the issue of abortion. Recommendation 6 of the Expert Group meeting stated:

Governments and intergovernmental and non-governmental organizations are urged to recognize that abortion is a major public health concern and one of the most neglected problems affecting women's lives. Women everywhere should have access to sensitive counselling and safe abortion services.

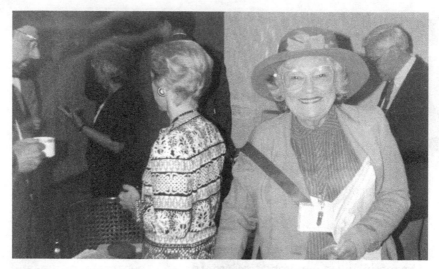

Bella Abzug, while I am talking to Steve Sinding on the U.S. delegation, 1994

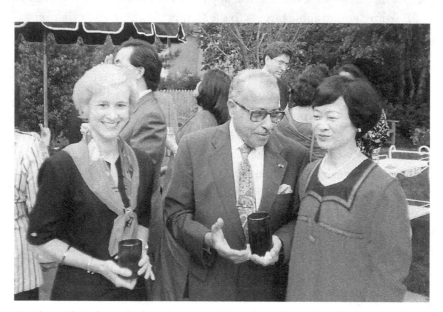

Meeting with Professor Mahran (center) and Mary Luke (right), VP of Programs at the
Centre for Development and Population Activities (CEDPA), 1994

Along with many others, I worked with Tim Wirth, former Senator from Colorado and the first U.S. Under Secretary of State for Global Affairs, on the preparations leading up to the Cairo Conference. I was appointed one of several team leaders of the 43-member U.S. delegation to ICPD (September 1994), under the leadership of Tim Wirth with Vice President Al Gore serving as the official head. For the first time, half of the members of the U.S. delegation were representatives of civil society, including a number of women's groups. Among the dynamic personalities was Bella Abzug, a prominent feminist and former congresswoman from New York. She regaled us each day with a colorful hat and rousing interventions during plenary sessions.

The 1994 ICPD was the largest international conference of its kind. There were over 11,000 registered participants representing governments, intergovernmental agencies, UN special agencies and organizations, non-governmental organizations (NGOs), and the media. An estimated 20,000 people gathered, under heavy security, in Cairo for this historic event. Egyptian President Mohamed Hosni Mubarak was president of the conference, and Dr. Maher Mahran, Minister of Population and Family Welfare of Egypt, served as the ex-officio vice president.

Among the delegates to the conference, there were over 1,200 NGOs from 138 countries. In addition, there was a parallel NGO Forum with over 4,200 representatives from more than 1,500 NGOs representing 133 countries. USAID and its cooperating agencies contributed significantly to the NGO Forum and helped ensure strong participation. Peggy Curlin, President of CEDPA, a USAID-funded NGO with a network of alumnae from 30 countries, played an important role in the NGO Forum as well as on the U.S. delegation. The conference also attracted 4,000 members of the media from around the world.

For the nine days of ICPD, there was a whirlwind of activity with people working late into the night and early morning hours. I served as a lead U.S. negotiator for five chapters of the ICPD Programme of Action, including the critical one on the resources required to implement the Cairo recommendations. In the process, I worked closely with leaders from Germany, which, at the time, was President of the European Union. I also had an opportunity to spend time with senior government and NGO officials from around the world as well as with Vice President Gore in several smaller U.S. delegation meetings.

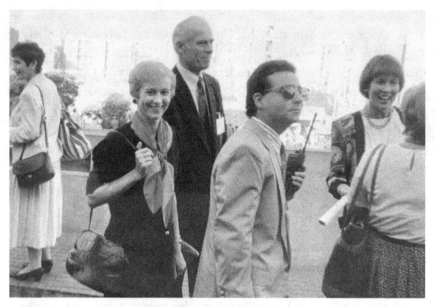

Arriving at the conference center in Cairo with Margaret Pollack (top right), ready for a long day and evening of meetings, 1994

One evening, members of the U.S. delegation and guests took a break and went on a cruise on the Nile where we were accompanied by Egyptian security boats. While admiring the sights of Cairo from this historic river, the longest in the world, I remember having a delightful conversation over drinks with Jane Fonda. We switched back and forth between English and French since we were both bilingual and loved France. An ardent feminist, Jane was at ICPD to advocate for the right of every woman to decide whether, when, and how many children to have and to enjoy full empowerment and equality. Jane was attending the conference with her husband Ted Turner, the founder of the cable news channel CNN.

The U.S. delegation, together with government and private sector leaders from around the world, helped shape the family planning and reproductive health agenda at ICPD, working in partnership with 178 other governments and with the active engagement of NGOs.

The most controversial issue under debate at ICPD was the language around abortion, with the delegation of the Holy See providing fierce opposition. The Vatican representatives managed to get a number of other country delegations to join them. However, for the first time, there was international recognition of the fact that unsafe abortion was one of the root causes of maternal mortality and morbidity around the world, with recommendations that "where abortion is not against the law, it should be safe." The Cairo Programme of Action further stipulated that women should have access to quality services for the management of the complications of unsafe abortion and that post-abortion counselling, education, and family planning should be offered to avoid repeat abortion. Unfortunately, due to the strong objections of the Holy See and the domestic politics in the United States and other countries, it was not possible to agree on a stron-

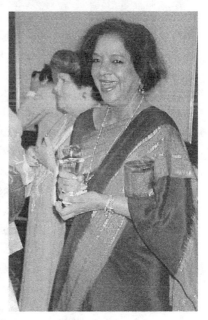

Dr. Nafis Sadik (center), Executive Director of UNFPA, and Peggy Curlin (left), President of CEDPA, 1994

ger statement about access to safe abortion as a human right and the imperative for governments to reform restrictive abortion laws.

Overall, the Cairo conference was a huge success due in large part to the pivotal roles of Dr. Nafis Sadik, Executive Director of UNFPA and Secretary-General of the ICPD, and Dr. Fred Sai, Chair of the Main Committee. The paradigm shift to "woman-centered" reproductive health care was the most significant outcome of the Cairo Conference. Indeed, comprehensive reproductive health was endorsed as a key component to protect women's health and the quality of life on this planet. As Dr. Sadik underscored in her closing comments at the conference, "I remain committed to building the future by building the power to choose."

IMPLEMENTING THE ICPD PROGRAMME OF ACTION

After ICPD, USAID's Office of Population took the lead in launching many new initiatives and expanded partnerships with women's and environmental groups, religious organizations, and other donors—governments, multilateral agencies, and U.S. foundations. We organized, together with the Population Council, a U.S./U.K.-sponsored Donors' Workshop on Implementing Reproductive Health Programs in New York in June 1995.

The most rewarding part of my tenure as Director was implementing the reproductive health mandate from ICPD while retaining a strong family planning focus. We launched several innovative programs leading up to the Cairo Conference, including one to improve family planning counselling, service delivery guidelines, and quality of care standards. The masterminds behind the Maximizing Access and Quality of Care (MAQ) initiative were Drs. Jim Shelton, Roy Jacobstein, and Jeff Spieler. In another bold action, we also started the Post-Abortion Care (PAC) program to treat complications of unsafe abortion while also offering family planning counselling and services.

The Office of Population developed new initiatives on gender, family planning, and women's empowerment; engaging men as partners; contraception and reproductive health needs of adolescents and young adults; and reduction of harmful practices such as female genital mutilation. Other areas of focus were supporting family planning and reproductive health initiatives in the private commercial sector and humanitarian organizations, addressing population and environment issues, treatment of sexually transmitted diseases and HIV prevention, as well as breastfeeding and increased linkages with safe motherhood. We ensured that reproductive health needs and interventions were incorporated into the Office of Population's broad portfolio of projects.

In 1999, I joined other delegates from around the world for a five-year review of progress in implementing the Cairo Programme of Action. I was a member of the U.S. delegation to the Hague Forum (February 1999) and the ICPD+5 Preparatory Committee (April 1999). In examining how far we had come since the Cairo conference, Barbara Crane, Dianne Sherman, and I prepared in early 1999 a comprehensive USAID report entitled *From Commitment to Action: Meeting the Challenges of ICPD.*

DEALING WITH LEGAL AND POLICY RESTRICTIONS

The 1990s was a period of great programmatic advances for USAID's population and reproductive health portfolio as well as unprecedented Congressional threats to a program aimed at saving and improving women's lives. We faced many challenges and constraints from the Newt Gingrich-led House of Representatives, which came into power in January 1995. Over the next few years, we had to deal with heavy Congressional harassment and additional legislative restrictions along with budget cuts and staff reductions. At the same time, we faced new and more cumbersome Agency systems and procedures.

Since joining USAID in 1977, I had managed to survive the Carter, Reagan, and George H. W. Bush eras as well as Republican and Democratic-controlled Houses of Congress. In 1984, the Mexico City policy was introduced by President Reagan, which prohibited overseas U.S. government-funded NGOs from performing or promoting abortion as a method of family planning, even with their own resources. Since then, every Democratic Administration has repealed the Mexico City policy (known as the Global Gag Rule), and it has been reinstated by Republican Administrations. The additional restrictions introduced by the Trump Administration have had the most far-reaching negative consequences.

I was fortunate to take over the Office of Population when President Clinton rescinded the Mexico City Policy two days after his inauguration. There was great jubilation among the staff. We immediately began preparing the necessary paperwork to refund the International Planned Parenthood Federation and the Human Reproduction Programme of the World Health Organization along with UNFPA. The whole process took several months given the number of reviews and signatures required.

There were other policies imposed by Congress that impacted USAID's population and reproductive health program, including the Helms Amendment, which was introduced in 1973. It prohibits the use of foreign assistance to pay for the performance of abortion as a method of family planning or to motivate or coerce any person to practice abortion. The Kemp-Kasten Amendment prohibits funding an organization or program, as determined by the U.S. president, which supports or participates in the management of a program of coercive abortion or involuntary sterilization. This has been applied by Republican Administrations to withhold funding from UNFPA because of its support to China. There is also Congressional language and program guidance to ensure voluntary use of family planning and reproductive health services and informed choice of contraceptive methods.

The biggest challenge during my tenure as Director of USAID's Office of Population was dealing with restrictions on the disbursement of funds imposed by the Republican majority in the House of Representatives. The initiative was fueled by Representative Chris Smith (R-NJ) in an effort to kill or severely cripple our program. The "metering" of funds meant that organizations supported by our office were only given small allotments of funds at a time throughout the year rather than a single disbursement. My deputy, Scott Radloff, created a master "metering" chart that helped keep all these programs functioning during this difficult period. Without his carefully crafted plan, some programs would have been unable to continue their critical activities. Eventually, these punitive Congressional restrictions were lifted.

Having sufficient funds to sustain our diverse program portfolio and respond to family planning and reproductive health needs in the developing world remained an ongoing concern. Pathfinder International, one of the office's largest grantees, paid for a full-page ad in *The New York Times* in July 1996, calling upon Congress to oppose funding cuts to international family planning programs. The ad appeared on the same day that Pathfinder received the United Nations Population Award for its outstanding contributions to increasing women's access to vital family planning and reproductive health services.

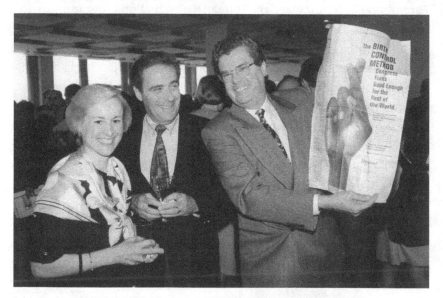

John Dumm, Senior Vice President of Pathfinder and former USAID colleague, showing Dr. Allan Rosenfield and me the famous *New York Times* ad, 1996

My USAID Colleagues

Although we worked in a huge and increasingly complex bureaucracy and had to deal with many internal as well as external obstacles, we always managed to find ways to maneuver through roadblocks and keep USAID's population and reproductive health program advancing.

I was fortunate to work in a close-knit environment where we shared a common vision and determination to make a difference in improving the lives of women and their families around the world. My colleagues were talented, hard-working, and deeply committed to expanding the impact of USAID's population assistance. They were also warm, enthusiastic, ingenious, and entertaining. Our Christmas parties, which featured hilarious skits, were renowned throughout the Agency.

Between meetings and work deadlines, I loved walking around and talking to staff to learn more about their accomplishments along with the challenges they faced. I welcomed everyone to stop by my office for a chat. My overseas trips to meet with USAID colleagues and partners and to see groundbreaking work in the field were always inspiring and energizing.

As Director, I was lucky to have exceptional deputies (Margaret Neuse, Gary Cook, and Scott Radloff) along with outstanding division chiefs and staff. There were so many other colleagues I admired and with whom I worked for many years, including Jim Shelton, Jeff Spieler, Roy Jacobstein, and my close friend and collaborator, Barbara Crane, just to mention a few.

By the 1990s, there were quite a few women who held important positions in our office as well as in other offices throughout the Agency, including in USAID missions around the world. It was very heartening to witness such a sea change and to have so many accomplished and delightful female colleagues and friends! Duff Gillespie remained my boss for 22 years, as each of us advanced. I valued his strategic vision, dedication, and amazing ability to get actions approved through the bureaucracy. I was also grateful for his mentorship and support of my taking on increasing responsibilities.

After working at USAID two decades longer than I had planned and having had an extremely rewarding career, despite the many bureaucratic and political frustrations, I was ready to move back to the private sector. In

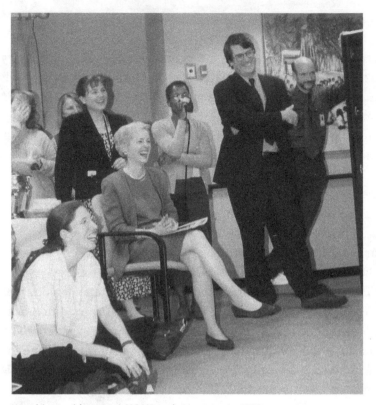

Watching a video at my USAID retirement party, 1999

June of 1999, my colleagues gave me a grand farewell party, orchestrated by Scott Radloff. There was a lot of roasting, toasting, exchange of fun gifts, skits, videos, songs, and laughter. I remember Duff noting in his remarks "How could someone so nice be so tough?!" I was very moved by the many tributes as well as being honored with the USAID *Distinguished Career Service Award.*

Most of all, it was an opportunity for me to express my deep gratitude for all the precious friendships I had developed over 22½ years and the many significant policy and programmatic advances we achieved as a global team. The successes were a result of strategic partnerships with governments and NGOs as well as with multilateral agencies, other donors, and the commercial sector.

I appreciate the continuing camaraderie with my former fellow Office Directors who are all remarkable people and served with distinction

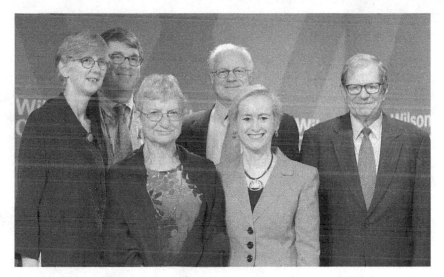

Current and former USAID Office of Population and Reproductive Health Directors at the Wilson Center, 2015: Ellen Starbird, Scott Radloff, Margaret Neuse, Duff Gillespie, Liz Maguire, Steve Sinding (left to right). THE WILSON CENTER

during their respective terms: Rei Ravenholt (1965–1978), Joe Speidel (1978–1983), Steve Sinding (1983–1986), Duff Gillespie (1986–1993), and, following my tenure (1993–1999), Margaret Neuse (2000–2006), and Scott Radloff (2006–2013) along with the current Director, Ellen Starbird. The one person I haven't seen in two decades is Rei Ravenholt, who was the genius behind the creation of USAID's global population assistance program.

The rest of us have kept in touch during the last 20 years and have enjoyed the chance to see each other whenever possible. After leaving USAID, my colleagues continued to make major contributions to the international family planning and reproductive health field, either serving as CEOs and/or in important positions in academia, as consultants, and on the Boards of non-profit organizations.

We formed close friendships around the work we did together for many years, the accomplishments during our tenures as Office Directors, as well as the political and other challenges we confronted. In 2008, Joe, Steve, Duff, Margaret, and I co-authored a report entitled *Making the Case for U.S. International Family Planning Assistance*.

We also celebrated together the 50th anniversary of USAID's population program in June 2015 with a panel session hosted by the Wilson Center: "Changing the World: How USAID's 50 Years of Family Planning has Transformed People, Economies, and the Planet."

In addition, four of us participated in a session called "Voices of Experience: A Conversation with Former Directors of USAID's Office of Population and Reproductive Health" in January 2018, hosted by the Center for Global Development in Washington, D.C. At these events, we reflected on the opportunities, progress, and threats USAID's population and reproductive health program faced during our tenures as director. Sadly, under the Trump Administration, the program is going through its most challenging period ever, while staff are continuing to do vital work around the world.

PART THREE

Fighting for Sexual and Reproductive Rights

LEADERSHIP OF IPAS

7

Enhancing Ipas's Presence and Impact

In early 1999, after 22 years at USAID, I heard from a good friend, Dr. Pouru Bhiwandi, that "The job of CEO of Ipas is open. You should do it!" At the time, Pouru was Chair of the Board of this international non-profit organization headquartered in Chapel Hill, North Carolina. I followed her advice and applied for the position. Two decades earlier, I had visited Ipas when it was a small operation and was impressed with its work.

Ipas was founded in 1973 with a unique mission: ending the needless deaths and injuries from unsafe abortion. Ipas later coined the word "comprehensive abortion care," which encompasses safe elective abortion, treatment of the complications of unsafe abortion, provision of family planning information and services, and referral for other reproductive health care.

When I received the offer to become CEO of Ipas, I accepted it without hesitation. This was my chance to focus on the one area of women's reproductive health and rights where USAID could not work due to Congressional restrictions. Throughout my travels in Africa, Asia, and Latin America, I witnessed huge needs in this neglected area and was a strong proponent of the right of every woman to make her own reproductive decisions free from fear or harm. I also looked forward to working more closely with Pouru, an esteemed Indian ob-gyn with an exuberant personality, and with other Board and staff members I knew.

I started at Ipas on September 1, 1999, feeling exhilarated and liberated! There were no layers of government bureaucracy, no Congressional constraints, and no legal limits on our work. At Ipas, there was complete freedom of speech and action. I was privileged to work on a critical mission with smart and dedicated staff, together with a supportive Board of Directors. Everyone was warm and welcoming, and I embraced my new family enthusiastically.

Ipas had about 100 employees, almost all based at headquarters. My overall goal as the new CEO was to safeguard the mission and culture of Ipas while increasing the organization's resources, size, visibility, geographic coverage, and impact. During the first six months, my highest priorities were to visit a couple of Ipas focus countries, spend time with all the staff, meet with major donors, and identify potential new funders. I also wanted to recruit additional talent on the Executive Team and the Board, and to develop a strategic framework around Ipas's mission.

A month after I arrived, I left on my first trip to Vietnam to see Ipas's work. Among those accompanying me were senior officials from two of our largest donors. This was one of the most fascinating trips during my tenure at Ipas. I spent time in both Ho Chi Minh City and Hanoi. I developed a better understanding of Ipas's critical role in training health care providers in safe abortion care and post-abortion family planning counselling and services, along with upgrading health facilities and the quality of care.

I was somewhat surprised to find my Vietnamese colleagues so welcoming considering the terrible devastation inflicted by the U.S. during the Vietnam War. One of the first people I met was a government official who began the conversation by asking my age. I was initially perplexed by this question. I learned, however, that my answer was important because it governed how she should address me. It turned out that we were nearly the same age.

I enjoyed getting to know our local Ipas staff and consultants along with other Vietnamese colleagues. It was also a chance to bond with members of our travelling group. The clinic visits and meetings with health officials were fascinating as were the historical landmarks we visited and all aspects of the local culture. A special highlight for me was seeing a uterine evacuation procedure for the first time performed by an Ipas-trained health care provider in a large, well-equipped hospital. From the standpoint of a tourist, I was excited to visit one of the world's most spectacular scenes—Halong Bay, located on the northeast coast, with emerald waters, grottoes, and giant limestone islands covered with rain forests.

OPENING NEW FRONTIERS

There was another important milestone in the fall of 1999 with the newly created Africa Alliance for Women's Reproductive Health and Rights. This initiative was led by Dr. Khama Rogo, a Kenyan ob-gyn and powerful activist for women's health. He served as Ipas's Vice President for Africa and Medical Affairs. In December, I joined Dr. Rogo and leaders from around Africa as well as selected Ipas staff and consultants at "The Summit at Mount Kenya." The purpose of the meeting was to conduct Ipas's first comprehensive planning exercise for Africa, outlining key strategies and action plans for the next five years. The African participants were mostly ob-gyns and mid-level health practitioners—all dedicated to increasing women's access to reproductive health care, including safe abortion.

The first evening, we gathered for an informal discussion where participants recounted their experiences dealing with abortion. These were powerful stories of personal transformation, which I will never forget. Many of the participants acknowledged that they were initially opposed to abortion. However, having seen women suffer and die needlessly from unsafe, illegal procedures, they changed their opinions. They all became eloquent advocates for a woman's right to control her fertility.

An overarching theme of the meeting was Ipas's role as a leader in advancing women's reproductive health and rights. Participants agreed that Ipas must serve as a risk-taker and address the three "U"s: unsafe sex, unwanted pregnancy, and unsafe abortion. As one of the African "visionaries" commented, "Ipas must shame leaders to give women the rights they deserve." In my remarks to the participants, I stated, "Each of us must leave here with renewed resolve to speak out on behalf of women's reproductive health and rights. We must help mobilize increased commitment and determination to deal with this critical, sensitive, and neglected frontier . . . . The challenges and opportunities we face are daunting. The time for action is now!"

After having inspired each other to take bold action, we enjoyed an evening game drive to see the wild animals in the reserve not far from our hotel, which straddled the equator. After admiring the many different species, we decided to adopt the giraffe as the Ipas mascot, since it is such a majestic animal, standing tall above all others, with great vision, wisdom, and courage.

When Dr. Rogo accepted a senior position at the World Bank in early 2001, I immediately called Dr. Eunice Brookman-Amissah. I had met her on a visit to Ghana when I was Director of USAID's Office of Population and she was Minister of Health. I saw her again at the April 1999 Cairo + 5 Conference in The Hague, where she was serving as the Ghanaian Ambassador to the Kingdom of the Netherlands. I reached Dr. Brookman-Amissah immediately upon her return to Accra after completing her service as Ambassador and before she had unpacked her bags. The stars were aligned when I managed to persuade her to become Ipas's Vice President for Africa, before she could even consider other exciting career options. Notably, Dr. Brookman-Amissah had served as Ipas's first Country Representative for Ghana during the period 1994–1996 and was an outspoken supporter of post-abortion care before she became Minister of Health.

Ambassador Dr. Brookman-Amissah assumed her new position at Ipas in June 2001. She served during the rest of my tenure as CEO and beyond as an eloquent and highly effective advocate throughout the region and around the world for women's sexual and reproductive health and rights. The Alliance became a powerful vehicle to build networks and partnerships throughout Africa. With limited resources, it provided peer support for brave pioneers and advocates who might otherwise have felt lonely speaking out on abortion issues in their own countries.

BUILDING THE EXECUTIVE TEAM

In my first few months, I began to assess needs on the Ipas Board and executive staff. I was thrilled when the person I most admired in the international reproductive health arena, Professor Mahmoud Fathalla of Egypt, accepted the invitation to become a Director of Ipas. Other well-known leaders in our field also served on the Board, as noted later.

In terms of executive staff, I felt extremely fortunate to have Ann Leonard as a colleague and confidante; she had served as acting CEO of Ipas before my arrival. She continued to oversee development, and training and service delivery improvement (TSDI) as well as the Regional Desk for Africa. Ann officially became my senior advisor beginning in early 2002 and was a member of the Executive Team. Ann had oversight of an increasingly broad portfolio, which encompassed, in addition to TSDI, technologies and clinical affairs and later youth. I have treasured her friendship and wise counsel both during and after I retired from Ipas. In my first few years at Ipas, Judith Winkler provided seasoned leadership of an expanded Information Services program, which included communications, the website, and the library. She also guided curriculum development and the work of the Desks for Latin America and the Caribbean (LAC) and Europe/North America.

I believed that Dr. Barbara Crane would make an excellent addition to my evolving Executive Team, given her extensive policy background as well as her skills in research, evaluation, and communications. I had worked closely with Barbara at USAID for most of the 1990s, including during the Cairo Conference and follow-up. I greatly valued her many technical contributions and high level of productivity as well as her close friendship. After several months of "wooing" her to Chapel Hill, I convinced Barbara to leave Washington, D.C. in the summer of 2000 and join Ipas. She did an exceptional job throughout my tenure, overseeing the Policy and Research and Evaluation units as well as other portfolios on a short-term basis. Barbara provided much-appreciated assistance on corporate communications, European donors, the Ipas Board, and indeed on almost every important issue.

Other key members joined my Executive Team in January 2002. Dr. Anu Kumar, formerly of WHO's Human Reproduction Programme and the MacArthur Foundation, took over the critical role of overseeing and expanding the development and communications areas, and later, Ipas's work on community engagement and mobilization. Anu is now providing outstanding leadership of Ipas as the current CEO.

For Executive Vice President of Programs, I hired Mary Luke, formerly of CEDPA and Planned Parenthood International Division where she served as Regional Director for Asia and the Pacific. She brought tremendous commitment, skills, and experience to this critical position, which included recruiting and overseeing the work of the Ipas Regional and Country Directors. This core team remained throughout my tenure, until Mary retired in May 2014 and Traci Baird took over, also providing outstanding leadership.

When I joined Ipas, John Dorward was doing a fantastic job covering finance, human resources, organizational development, information technology, and manufacturing and quality assurance. He stepped down as Chief Operating Officer at the end of 2002 after 23 years of distinguished service. It was impossible to find someone of John's dedication, experience, and tireless efforts to cover such a large portfolio. There were several individuals who filled the important position of Executive Vice President of Finance and Administration during my tenure. However, one of the challenges I faced was finding the right profile of qualified people with a passion for Ipas's mission, culture, and global staff, together with previous relevant experience with an international non-profit organization. Mike Florio held this position before I retired. I appreciated his expertise and warm personality.

STRATEGIC PLANNING

In the fall of 1999, I was anxious to begin development of a new results framework so that Ipas could better measure and track its impact. This was essential in reporting to donors on the value they received for their investment. We also needed a results framework in order to take appropriate corrective measures and make continuous improvements. I was delighted when another great leader in our field, Dr. Amy Tsui, who was Director of the Carolina Population Center at UNC-Chapel Hill, graciously offered to provide technical assistance in this important exercise. I had known Amy when I was at USAID, and she first became Project Director of the MEASURE Evaluation program, another post-Cairo USAID initiative. The results framework that emerged was the first of several iterations during my tenure. I was extremely grateful to Amy for her early support and later convinced her to join the Ipas Board. She offered valuable expertise and insights, including in her role as Chair.

Beginning in 2000, the Ipas mission had a dual focus around two closely interrelated goals: *reduce maternal deaths and injuries due to unsafe abortion, and advance women's sexual and reproductive rights*. We developed regional strategic plans for Africa and Latin America, followed by other regional strategies and country action plans.

Over the years, we designed new and more comprehensive organizational results frameworks and plans. In the last five-year strategic plan before I retired, Ipas's stated purpose had evolved to: *Enhance the ability and rights of women, including young women, to obtain comprehensive abortion care and prevent unwanted pregnancy.* The plan had three major outputs: ensuring that comprehensive abortion care, including contraception, was "fully integrated into organized health systems"; women had "the knowledge, skills, social support, and sources of care in their communities to make and act upon their reproductive decisions"; and there was "a supportive policy, legislation, and rights environment to achieve Ipas's goals." There was a fourth output on being an "effective and efficient organization demonstrating innovation and leadership."

FUNDRAISING

Upon my arrival, I talked to Ipas's traditional donors to express my appreciation for their sustained support and to share my vision for the future. I was especially grateful for the funding from a large anonymous donor as well as from the Packard, Hewlett, and other U.S. foundations. With the help of a terrific team, I launched a campaign to raise additional funds from U.S. donors as well as from European governments so that we could expand Ipas's geographic footprint and results.

Ipas had a small amount of USAID funds as a sub-contractor on a training contract on post-abortion care. However, the situation changed when George W. Bush was sworn in as President in January 2001. When he reinstated the Mexico City policy (the Global Gag Rule), I decided, in consultation with the Board and key staff, that Ipas would withdraw from USAID funding. We could not impose unethical restrictions on overseas organizations working legally in their own countries to address women's reproductive health needs. Ipas's core belief was that no woman should have to risk her life or health to end an unwanted pregnancy. Our decision was respected by all our donors and partners.

A top personal priority as CEO was to build partnerships with as many

European donors as possible who shared a deep commitment to Ipas's mission. At the ICPD+5 conference in 1999, there was a breakthrough on abortion. Language in paragraph 63iii of the report stated: *In circumstances where abortion is not against the law, health systems should train and equip health service providers and take other measures to ensure that such abortions are safe and accessible. Additional measures should be taken to safeguard women's health.* Ipas took the initiative to operationalize this language and began to move beyond a predominant focus on post-abortion care in earlier years to supporting comprehensive abortion care to the full extent of the law.

Working closely with Barbara Crane, we developed concept papers for major European government donors, recognizing the potential for their financial assistance as they were not encumbered by the political limitations that prevented U.S. government support for safe abortion. Ipas had previously received modest funding from the U.K., Sweden, and the Netherlands on which we could build. We started with colleagues from the U.K. Department for International Development (DFID), whom we had known from the 1994 ICPD in Cairo, as well as from the Ministries for Foreign Affairs in Sweden and Finland. All three governments funded an Ipas global initiative on *Advancing Access to Safe Abortion*. This was designed to translate the ICPD+5 language into action and expand programs especially in Africa and South Asia.

We also developed a close partnership with Elly Leemhuis-de Regt at the Dutch Ministry of Foreign Affairs who responded with a grant to Ipas. We later secured funding from Norway, followed by Denmark and Germany. Merrill Wolf on our Ipas team became a valuable collaborator in working with the European donors, as did several Country Directors.

Our trips to European capitals to meet with donors were almost entirely focused on work, with little or no time to sightsee. There were a couple of exceptions. In April 2010, when Barbara and I were visiting officials in The Hague, the Eyjafjallajökull volcano in Iceland erupted, ejecting volcanic ash over a large part of Europe and shutting down air traffic. During a couple of days of visiting museums and taking a side trip to the picturesque city of Delft, we pursued various ways to get back to the U.S. with increasing concern as major airports in northern Europe closed one by one. We were lucky to identify a flight that would depart from Barcelona for Atlanta. A major problem we encountered was that the trains were on strike in France. Since there were no rental cars available, Barbara and I hired a cousin of our hotel's concierge to drive us. On the two-day trip from The Hague all the way to Barcelona, we travelled 1,000 miles, enjoying wonderful scenes of springtime in the Dutch, Belgian, French, and Spanish countryside. We arrived with a day to spare before our flight, allowing us time to stroll through Barcelona's old city, visit the Picasso Museum, and eat lunch on the waterfront.

Near the end of my tenure, several Ipas colleagues and I opened a dialogue with the French government to support Ipas's growing work in Francophone Africa. Leila Hessini and Kat Turner joined me on a memorable "hardship" trip to Paris. In addition to enjoying the "City of Light" and fine cuisine, we discussed with government and NGO officials Ipas's mission, the unmet needs, and the opportunities for expanded work in French-speaking countries in West Africa. We received a warm reception from our French colleagues who expressed an interest in Ipas's programs and the possibilities for collaboration. We were especially appreciative of the facilitative role of Thomas Dubois of the French Ministry of Foreign Affairs.

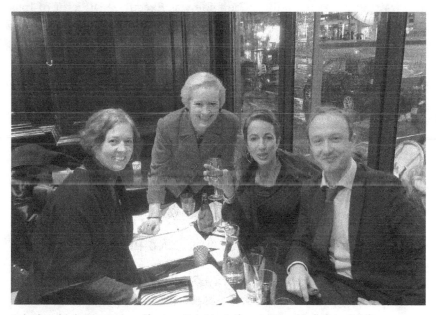

Enjoying drinks in a Paris café, 2014: Kat, Liz, Leila, and Thomas (left to right)

The European donor partnerships proved vital in expanding Ipas's resources over the years, as did the major support we received from a large anonymous donor, together with funding from other traditional donors and a growing number of U.S. foundations. All these donors were committed to addressing unsafe abortion as a major cause of high maternal mortality and morbidity and to expanding women's access to safe care. They were generous in providing new or increased funding for Ipas.

Throughout my tenure, fundraising remained one of my core responsibilities. What I enjoyed most about my meetings with donors was discussing Ipas's success stories as well as challenges in the external environment. It was easy to make the case for how we could expand our reach, innovation, and impact with more resources.

I was fortunate that Ipas had a first-rate team of experts devoted to fundraising and all that this effort entails. In my first couple of years as CEO, Ann Leonard continued to lead the development team, with Roxanne Henderson serving as her deputy. As soon as Anu Kumar joined Ipas at the beginning of 2002, she became actively engaged in fundraising and provided strategic guidance and oversight of the entire development effort. Katie Early was a long-time, pivotal player in the organization's fundraising work, including when she was Executive Director of Ipas beginning in the mid-1980s. Working under Anu, Katie became Director of Development and continued to expand the group of committed, experienced development officers. The development team worked hard on cultivating and supporting current institutional donors, increasing support from multilateral and bilateral donors, and prospecting for new foundation and individual donors. They also kept busy preparing an ever-increasing number of detailed proposals and reports, totaling almost 150 in my final year. In addition, Ipas launched a major gifts program, under Annie O'Leary. I greatly appreciated the tireless efforts of the entire development team and was proud of all their accomplishments.

GROWING IPAS'S COUNTRY OFFICES AND PROGRAMS

As Ipas's annual budget increased each year, we were able to strengthen and expand major areas of work and especially Ipas's presence and activities in each region.

We made a concerted effort to recruit local highly qualified staff in priority countries in Latin America, Africa, and Asia. When I joined Ipas, there was a strong Ipas office in Mexico and a few other small country offices. As our resources grew, we converted Ipas consultants into full-time staff in key countries as well as recruited new Country Directors. I was committed to having all local staff, including directors, in our focus countries. This distinguished Ipas from some of our colleague organizations who used expatriates at the time to head at least a few of their country programs.

local staff as leads.

In addition to the pivotal leadership roles played by Mary Luke, Executive Vice President for Programs, and Dr. Eunice Brookman-Amissah, Vice President for Africa, we were fortunate to have a series of outstanding Regional Directors. Overseeing the Country Directors and programs in the Latin America region was Virginia Chambers followed later by Christopher Bross. Jennifer Potts, Uche Ekenna, Iqbal Hossain, and William Sampson, at different times, served in this role for Africa. During my tenure, there were several Regional Directors for Asia, including Don Weeden, Traci Baird, Wendy Darby, Amin Islam, and Karen Otsea, with Mary Luke filling in, as needed.

We also had relatively small programs in the U.S. and Europe for a number of years, focused on training and equipping health care providers in comprehensive abortion care and ensuring access to appropriate technologies. Traci Baird provided oversight of this work, aided by Rivka Gordon and later Donna Ruscavage serving as U.S. Program/Country Director.

The Ipas Country Directors came from diverse backgrounds. Their expertise ranged from training, public health, and maternal and child health care, to social and economic development, poverty reduction, advocacy, women's rights, communications, marketing, and program management. These leaders had previous valuable experience working for local non-governmental organizations, international agencies, governments, and donors. All the Country Directors were united in their deep commitment to Ipas's mission and work. They were excellent strategists and passionate spokespeople, dealing skillfully with politically and culturally sensitive issues. Given the heavy workload, each director was generally paired with a strong manager to help provide oversight of the staff and office operations.

During my tenure, Ipas Country Directors from Latin America included: Eliana del Pozo and Dr. Malena Morales of Bolivia; Dr. Leila Adesse of Brazil; Andrea Saldaña Rivera, Dr. Nadine Gasman, and Dr. Raffaela Schiavon of Mexico; and Marta María Blandón of Nicaragua who guided Ipas's work in Central America since 1991. In Africa, we were fortunate to have: Saba Kidanemariam of Ethiopia; Dr. Koma Jehu-Appiah of Ghana; Dr. Sarah Onyango, Dr. Joachim Osur, and Erick Yegon of Kenya; Godfrey Kangaude and Chrispine Sibande of Malawi; Dr. Ejike Oji, Dr. Nihinlola Mabogunje, and Hauwa Shekarau of Nigeria; Valerie Tucker of Sierra Leone; Khosi Xaba, Mosotho Gabriel, and Karen Trueman of South Africa; and Felicia Sakala of Zambia. For the Asia region, we had outstanding Country Directors as well: S.M. Shahidullah of Bangladesh; V.S. Chandrashekhar and Vinoj Manning of India; Dr. Ni Ni of Myanmar; Dr. Indira Basnett of Nepal; Amina Mazhar and Ghulam Shabbir of Pakistan; and Do Thi Hong Nga of Vietnam. Those serving as director of the Ipas Africa Alliance, under the guidance of Dr. Brookman-Amissah, included Mosotho Gabriel and Dr. Joachim Osur. I salute all these inspirational leaders along with the Ipas staff who supported them!

The Ipas Country Directors and teams provided technical and financial assistance not only to Ministries of Health and private providers but also to national associations of obstetricians and gynecologists as well as midwives, legal and advocacy groups, and other civil society organizations, including women's, community, youth, and human rights groups, among others. They worked on building the capacity of public sector health systems to provide comprehensive, woman-centered abortion care and contraception. Scaling up training and equipping of health care providers, especially mid-level providers, was a key focus. In addition, the teams supported work at the community level and addressed the needs of adolescents and young adults along with policy, advocacy, and research initiatives.

The leaders of our country programs all had tough jobs. They worked long hours in challenging environments. There was always opposition to abortion, even though it was legal under at least certain circumstances in almost all Ipas focus countries. As an international organization, the Ipas

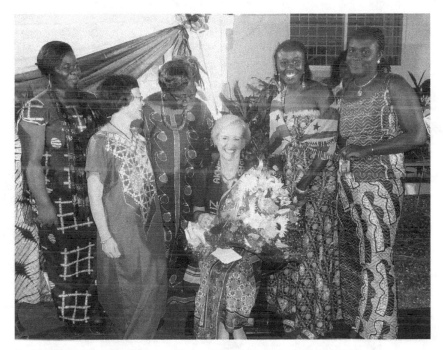

A party at the Ipas office in Accra, Ghana, 2007: Mary Luke (left) and Liz Maguire (seated). IPAS

country offices offered a wealth of expertise and creativity. We ensured that their experiences were shared within and between the regions as well as with the Chapel Hill office.

The most rewarding part of my job as CEO was visiting the Ipas country offices, spending time with staff and partners. I developed close friendships with the Country Directors and would have loved to have interacted with them on a weekly basis.

Everywhere I travelled, from Mexico to Kenya to India to Vietnam and many countries in between, I received a warm welcome and learned a great deal, enjoying my conversations with women and health care providers in urban and rural areas. I was always impressed with the dedication of everyone working on this common mission along with the innovative activities I witnessed. On every trip I wished that Ipas had greatly expanded resources to support many more people in need. Nevertheless, the assistance we provided was gratefully received.

During my overseas travels, I accumulated an abundance of unfor-

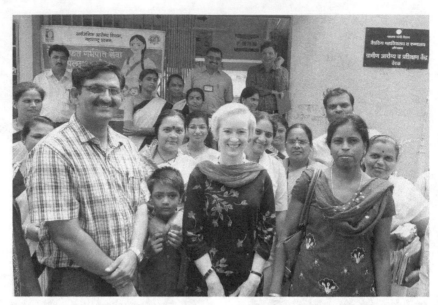

Visiting Corporation Hospital in Aurangabad, India, 2013. © Ipas Development Foundation (IDF)

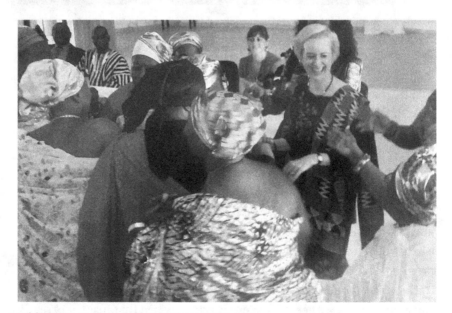

With Queen Mothers in eastern Ghana, 2010. Ipas

gettable experiences. One of these was seeing the pioneering work Ipas was doing with Queen Mothers in Ghana. These traditional community leaders of royal lineage, who number approximately 10,000 across the country, wield considerable power and play a critical role in helping to improve the health, education, and well-being of the women and families they serve. Ipas worked closely and effectively with Queen Mothers in support of their efforts to increase awareness and use of modern contraception and safe, legal abortion. On two different trips, I joined gatherings of the Queen Mothers in eastern Ghana. It was fascinating to hear them talk about their work and the issues of greatest concern in their communities, including women's ability to control their fertility. Following our discussions, I joined in the dancing and enjoyed the many hugs.

[handwritten margin note: partner w/ local leaders ↓ redefine. norms]

Another memorable experience was visiting northern Nigeria, a sharp contrast to eastern Ghana. That trip gave me a glimpse into what it was like to be a woman in a very conservative Muslim society. To show respect, I wore a head scarf, long-sleeved blouse, and skirt covering my legs. During my time in Kano, however, I made the mistake of trying to shake the hand of the director of one of the local hospitals. He did not reciprocate, and I quickly realized that I had breached protocol.

We visited a few health facilities in the city, including one large hospital that was operating with no running water. Afterwards, we toured a nearby rural area. With our local Ipas colleagues, I talked to several women living in one of the compounds that dotted the countryside. We were reminded that women could not leave their compound, even for a medical emergency, without the permission of their husbands. In this area, Ipas was supporting an outreach effort by local midwives and community workers to talk to women about their health needs and gain the approval of their husbands so that they could visit the nearest clinic to obtain family planning and other critical services. One of the midwives commented on the many challenges she faced working in this setting.

8

TECHNICAL LEADERSHIP
AND INNOVATIONS

From the beginning of my tenure, a top priority was to continue to enhance Ipas's technical leadership and innovation. When I arrived, I was thrilled to find outstanding technical directors in Chapel Hill, including Joan Healy (Training and Service Delivery Improvement), Janie Benson (Research, Monitoring, and Evaluation), and Charlotte Hord Smith (Policy and Advocacy). Midway through my term, Leila Hessini, whom I had first met in 1993 at USAID and later brought to Ipas, moved from serving as a senior Ipas policy advisor to become Director of Community Engagement and Mobilization. Marty Jarrell became head of the communications unit. These exceptionally committed and talented leaders built strong teams around them and worked effectively with the Country Directors. Ipas's technical directors were strategic, pioneering, and results driven. With their strong communications and cross-cultural skills, they were able to build successful partnerships and networks around the world.

ENHANCING HEALTH SYSTEM ACCESS

Under Joan Healy's direction, Ipas played a vital leadership role globally, regionally, and at the country level in increasing the quality, availability, and sustainability of comprehensive abortion care, including post-abortion care and contraception. Joan and other Ipas staff made significant contributions to the development of the first WHO safe abortion guidance in 2003 and subsequent revisions. Ipas was, in turn, tasked by WHO with helping to disseminate widely each set of guidelines and to assist national ministries of health in implementing them.

Our experts pioneered improved training strategies and techniques. They developed new curricula and training tools as well as standards and guidelines for woman-centered comprehensive abortion care. All these represented the state of the art and were used by Ipas and partner organizations. Ipas leaders were instrumental in getting safe abortion care incorporated into global standards for ob-gyns and mid-level providers and in their pre-service training in many countries. In addition, Joan and her colleagues helped Ipas country teams in their efforts to increase the effectiveness of health care providers and intervention sites. They focused on the primary level of the health system that was most accessible to underserved women. Ipas staff implemented new approaches for selecting, supporting, monitoring, and following up trained providers and service sites to ensure excellent care and the availability of reproductive health commodities. All these initiatives, including the many articles and documents published, expanded the evidence base for policy and program improvement.

quality ↑ care of primary facilities ↓ since 1st point of access to health system

Other innovations were the creation of a Global Trainers' Network, headed by Kat Turner, as well as the development of Values Clarification and Attitude Transformation (VCAT). This tool has been used effectively with health care providers and other stakeholders so that they could assess their core values and attitudes towards abortion. Everyone receiving VCAT training was better able to appreciate the consequences for women and adolescents who did not have access to the information and care they needed to make their own reproductive decisions. The use of VCAT helped establish better alignment between behavior, actions, and values. Ipas was a leader, working with other partners, in conducting VCAT workshops in many countries around the world.

IMPROVING QUALITY OF CARE

An important foundation for Ipas's work with national health systems was ensuring clinical accuracy, currency, and high standards of care. We were fortunate to have Dr. Laura Castleman, a well-known and admired ob-gyn, serve as Ipas Medical Director. She developed a Clinical Affairs team of staff and consultants, under the direction of Dr. Dalia Brahmi, another great Ipas hire, working with Bill Powell, Dr. Alice Mark, and others. One of their mandates was to provide up-to-date clinical information based on a careful review of the latest evidence along with standards and guidance to field staff. The *Clinical Updates in Reproductive Health* were widely appreciated by Ipas partners as well.

The Clinical Affairs team focused on compliance, building staff capacity, promoting performance and quality improvement initiatives, monitoring and reporting serious adverse events, and providing technical support to country teams and service delivery sites. They also conducted research and disseminated key findings. Ipas clinical staff worked closely with several key partner organizations, including WHO, the International Federation of Gynecology and Obstetrics, Gynuity Health Projects, the International Planned Parenthood Federation, and Marie Stopes International.

Engaging in Humanitarian Settings

Thanks to the commitment and hard work, especially of Joan Healy, Bill Powell, and Tam Fetters, Ipas became actively engaged in the Inter-Agency Working Group on Reproductive Health in Crises (IAWG). They advocated successfully for the inclusion of abortion in the *IAWG Field Manual for Reproductive Health in Conflict Settings* and participated in its dissemination.

Refugees and women in war-torn areas are especially vulnerable to sexual violence and rape and need ready access to care for the prevention and treatment of unwanted pregnancies. Ipas's efforts in humanitarian settings to train health care providers, provide updated guidelines, and ensure access to safe abortion care technologies have expanded substantially in recent years.

Increasing Community Access

An essential complement to Ipas's work with health systems during my tenure was helping women in communities gain access to the reproductive health information and services and social support they needed. This involved working closely with community health workers and organizations, including women's groups, as well as supporting local change agents to help women overcome barriers such as lack of knowledge about services, limited access to care, misinformation, fear, and stigma.

As this area obtained more resources, we created in September 2008 the Reaching Women Directly unit in Chapel Hill, under the dynamic leadership of Leila Hessini. The unit was renamed Community Engagement and Mobilization and later Community Access. Leila and her growing team of experts continued work on strategic alliances with feminist, human rights, and social justice networks as well as engaged mid-level health providers at a local, regional, and global level. They supported Ipas country offices in their expanding community-based initiatives and prepared a variety of tools and resources along with a theoretical framework for monitoring and evaluating the impact of this work. In 2009, Ipas organized a global community outreach meeting to build capacity among Ipas staff and partners from all developing regions.

Activities in Ipas focus countries included community assessments to determine knowledge, attitudes, and practices regarding SRHR and designing interventions to respond to the needs identified. Staff piloted new communications tools and strategies to reach women directly, using different media: radio, TV, billboards, websites, hotlines, YouTube videos, and posters, etc. They also engaged with local influential networks and leaders, such as the Queen Mothers in Ghana. Our programs in Ghana, Nigeria, and Zambia even conducted sensitization workshops on SRHR for police officers. This initiative was successful in diminishing police harassment and stigma around abortion as well as making it easier for women to obtain the reproductive health care they needed.

Another creative step was the use of mHealth mobile devices to educate women on where to access reproductive health information and services. In South Africa, for example, Ipas worked with a local non-profit organization using SMS messages to inform communities, including providers and clients, about medical abortion.

In Brazil, there was a particularly effective media campaign entitled *Know Your Rights* where victims of sexual violence could call a government hotline to learn about legal abortion and how to access services. Another powerful promotional video was entitled *Think about it* aimed at helping people think differently about abortion. This video was adapted for use in several other countries in the region.

In Nepal, I witnessed a successful initiative where female community health volunteers were trained to perform early pregnancy tests for women who wanted them and make referrals, as appropriate, to the nearest health facility. In another Ipas-supported project, nearly 1,000 women factory workers received training on sexual and reproductive health and rights. Some of these workers then became change agents in their communities.

Work at the community level became an increasingly high priority within Ipas's broad portfolio, resulting in technical and financial support to hundreds of local community-based organizations. Innovative activities and research were conducted in each Ipas country, with best practices and lessons learned shared across the organization.

One of Ipas's pivotal contributions was working with pharmacies and drug sellers at the community level to facilitate increased availability and use by women of medical abortion information and drugs. Ipas was a pioneer in this area, working with other local and international NGO partners.

not only work w/ doctors but also pharmacies

Ipas supported another groundbreaking approach—the harm-reduction model, initiated in Uruguay, where women could access pre- and post-abortion counselling services within the public health sector, while obtaining medical abortion drugs at pharmacies. This model was used to link women to networks of providers in countries where abortion was legally restricted.

FOCUSING ON THE NEEDS OF YOUNG PEOPLE

Along with the expansion of community-based activities, Ipas began to focus more on meeting the needs of youth. Staff tested creative ways of reaching adolescents and young people with information and services, working with youth organizations and medical student associations in addition to community-based networks. In 2003, Ipas Mexico launched a two-year process of examining youth needs and perspectives by conducting workshops with Ipas curriculum entitled *Gender or Sex: Who Cares?* Later, I had an opportunity to observe a sex education class at a public school in Mexico City. I was struck by the comprehensiveness of the approach, in sharp contrast to what was happening in U.S. public schools at the time.

In 2009, Ipas completed a global youth strategy, under Leila's direction, and expanded efforts to remove barriers for young women to understand their sexual and reproductive rights and gain access to contraception and safe abortion, especially medical abortion. Projects in different Ipas countries focused on strengthening interactive peer education, reaching both young women and men through trained youth leaders and peer educators in villages and towns. We considered it essential to work with men and boys as partners in supporting the rights of women and girls to prevent and manage safely unintended pregnancy.

In each Ipas country, model youth-friendly services were introduced, evaluated, and scaled up, with appropriate modifications. Young people were involved in the design and implementation of services to ensure that their specific sexual and reproductive health needs were being addressed. Building strong relationships between peer educators and local providers was key.

There were effective means of reaching thousands of young people with SRHR information—in popular radio broadcasts and street dramas as well as hotlines and text messages. In Nepal, for example, a national radio program, broadcast in every district in the country, included episodes about youth sexual and reproductive health. In Bolivia and Ghana, we provided support to young radio hosts talking about these issues.

Each Ipas country developed information materials, including leaflets, posters, and flipcharts to support youth mobilizers. A few countries experimented with youth-friendly "help points" in selected schools and universities. I visited one of these during a trip to Ethiopia and was pleased to see that students valued this service and the link provided to the nearest health facility.

Ipas published literature reviews on young women's abortion needs, experiences, and strategies as well as tools for use in safe abortion programming for youth. There were also articles and publications that advanced the state of the art, including ones focused on key issues of sexual violence and unwanted pregnancy.

We introduced a youth focus in all areas of Ipas's work, underscoring that this was an organization-wide priority. In taking this action, we highlighted the importance of respectful, confidential, and accessible care for young people. We also made a special effort to develop youth leaders in sexual and reproductive health and rights. The aim was to provide them with knowledge and skill building so that they could advocate on their own behalf as well as participate in national, regional, and global conferences on these critical issues. Ipas had an impressive group of young leaders on staff, including Laura Villa, Evelina Börjesson, Sarah Packer, Anisha Aggarwal (in India), and Cecilia Espinoza, among many others who participated in key regional and international meetings.

Later in my tenure, Karah Fazekas Pedersen took over as head of this important portfolio, joined by Ana Aguilera who was a dynamic addition to the team. Cecilia Espinosa and others continued to play key roles. They coordinated closely with and supported the activities of Ipas's country programs.

ADDRESSING STIGMA

Under the leadership of Leila Hessini and Anu Kumar, Ipas launched in 2009 an initiative to examine and address abortion stigma. Over the next several years, Ipas conducted pioneering research and developed and tested a tool for measuring abortion stigma at the individual and community level. Leila and Anu co-hosted abortion stigma webinars and co-authored an issue on abortion stigma in the journal *Stigma Research and Action*. Staff also produced and disseminated a promotional video entitled *Because abortion stigma affects us all*.

Ipas co-hosted a Bellagio Expert Group meeting in June 2012 with scholars, practitioners, and advocates from 11 countries from all regions to discuss work on abortion stigma and agree on a research and action agenda.

In 2014, the International Network for the Reduction of Abortion Discrimination and Stigma (INROADS) was launched, with Ipas playing the lead coordinating role. Since then, this initiative has grown dramatically and now includes members representing over 95 countries and 800 organizations. It is having an important impact on breaking down barriers and the discrimination and stigma associated with abortion, through sharing information, tools, stories, and other activities.

BUILDING SUSTAINABLE ACCESS TO REPRODUCTIVE HEALTH TECHNOLOGIES

Manual vacuum aspiration (MVA): Without safe and effective technologies, including contraceptives and abortion, there would be no comprehensive family planning and abortion care programs. Following the passage of the Helms Amendment to the U.S. Foreign Assistance Act in 1973, which prohibited USAID from continuing its abortion work, Ipas was created and charged with the further development and distribution of MVA instruments. MVA is a very simple, safe, and cost-effective technology used for uterine evacuation, miscarriage management, post-abortion care, and endometrial biopsy. As the organization grew, Ipas continued to serve as the leader in the manufacture, widespread distribution, and promotion of the latest abortion technologies.

Soon after I started as CEO, it was time to invest in upgrading the instruments so that they would be even simpler to use, more versatile, and easier to disinfect and sterilize. We were able to secure donor support for the research and development work. John Dorward and Gil Barner were central players in the first few years. Ann Leonard, working with others, provided outstanding leadership and expert guidance throughout this multi-year process, overcoming challenges along the way.

Thirty years after the initial completion of MVA instruments, Ipas introduced in 2003 the *Ipas EasyGrip Cannulae®* and in the following year the *Ipas MVA Plus®*. The design improvements represented the latest innovations in this remarkable technology and the state of the art in infection prevention. The new instruments were heat resistant for the first time so they could be sterilized by autoclave as well as by liquid chemical solutions. These upgrades made it easier for health care providers performing uterine evacuation in a wide variety of hospital settings as well as in urban and rural clinics around the world. Ipas produced useful materials about the proper use, processing, and cleaning of the new and improved instruments. While there are cheaper versions of manual vacuum aspiration instruments, the *Ipas MVA Plus®* remains a leading high-quality device.

When I joined Ipas, MVA instruments were still being manufactured and assembled, mostly by hand, in a small building on the main street of Carrboro, the adjacent community to Chapel Hill. As we scaled up our efforts, we outsourced the manufacturing of MVA instruments to a company in Taiwan. Ipas's strategy was to increase access to manual vacuum aspiration through engaging a wide network of distributors to reach health care providers in the public and private sectors around the world.

In 2009, Ipas took another bold step to expand the distribution of the latest MVA and other reproductive health technologies by launching a non-profit subsidiary, WomanCare Global (WCG). Ann Leonard and I recruited Saundra Pelletier to lead this new organization that assumed responsibility for manufacturing oversight, quality control, distribution, and marketing of MVA globally, under a subcontract agreement with Ipas. The new entity was registered as a U.K. charity known as WomanCare Global International (WCGI).

During the subsequent five years, we overcame "bumps in the road" and felt that Ipas benefitted overall from this process. We were able to reallocate to programmatic activities the substantial resources Ipas had expended previously on reproductive health technologies. In 2013, WCGI became independent from Ipas and entered into a strategic alliance with Evofem, a U.S.-based biotechnology company. Since 2017, the Ipas MVA instruments are being distributed by DKT WomanCare Global.

Medical abortion (MA): Early in my tenure, we also began to explore how Ipas could help women access medical abortion. This was a revolutionary technology, using pharmaceuticals—mifepristone in a combined regimen with misoprostol, or misoprostol alone. For the first time, women could have a choice of either MVA or MA, both safe and effective methods for uterine evacuation. The initial hurdle we faced was ensuring that MA could be registered and made affordable in countries where Ipas was working.

We adopted MA as a strategic focus of Ipas's work beginning in 2001 and formed an internal Medical Abortion Task Force. Ipas became a founding member of the International Consortium for Medical Abortion (ICMA) and served on the steering committee. Over the next 10 years, we integrated MA into all aspects of Ipas's work, including building clinical and training skills along with technical and programmatic capacity. We developed training curricula, counselling, and service delivery guidelines on MA, as well as fact sheets and educational materials for providers and women. As noted earlier, we trained different levels of health care professionals as well as pharmacists and conducted operations research on increasing the acceptability, accessibility, and use of medical abortion.

All this work—along with new projects, resources, and publications—increased under a global medical abortion initiative headed by Traci Baird during the period 2006–2011. Medical abortion was introduced in a growing number of low-resource settings in Africa, Asia, and Latin America, and our team began to devote time to addressing issues of MA drug access and sustainable supply. Ipas country programs launched innovative projects to make MA more widely known and available, including reaching women directly with information and support, using community outreach workers and pharmacists. India was one of the pioneering countries engaged in scaling up the use of MA, along with Mexico, Nepal, and Ethiopia, to mention a few.

Ipas became a "learning" environment for MA, exchanging knowledge, strategies, and lessons learned across the organization and with partners. Ipas India created MAPNet, a network of private providers to promote exchange of information and experiences using MA. This successful initiative was done in partnership with the Federation of Obstetric and Gynaecological Societies of India (FOGSI). Our Ipas team contributed to building the evidence base globally for the provision of medical abortion. We collaborated closely with Dr. Beverly Winikoff and her staff at Gynuity Health Projects who were the major trailblazers in this field, documenting that MA was safe for women's self-use. A growing number of organizations embraced this new technology and dramatically increased their work in this area. Ipas colleagues were active in national and regional networks that were formed as well as in a series of important conferences where participants discussed findings of major studies, best practices, challenges, and recommendations for future actions.

Over the years, there have been many advances in medical abortion, and it remains a very popular and widely used method. In every Ipas-supported country, MA increasingly became women's preferred method. The opportunity for self-use helped women overcome legal and policy restrictions, although barriers of cost, stigma, and accessibility still pose challenges in many areas. Moreover, to ensure women's full access to safe abortion care, including the treatment of complications of unsafe abortion, all major methods of uterine evacuation must be available to women and providers.

Contraceptives: Another high priority for Ipas and partners was to continue working with ministries of health and the commercial sector in Africa, Asia, and Latin America to build sustainable supplies of contraceptives and other reproductive health commodities. These are essential to effective programs and to protect the right of all women and girls to have safe reproductive choices.

9

POLICY AND ADVOCACY

The second major arm of Ipas's mission and work, in addition to expanding the quality, availability, and affordability of comprehensive abortion care, has been action in the policy and advocacy arena. At the country level, as well as in global and regional fora, Ipas became a fearless leader and the "go-to" organization in advocating for women's sexual and reproductive health and rights, including the right to safe and legal abortion. Ipas priorities included supporting local efforts to reform restrictive policies and guard against setbacks, contributing to the policy and regulatory frameworks to help women gain access to reproductive health care as allowed by local law, and advocating to improve the regional and global environment for women's fundamental rights. The support of European donors, WHO, and eventually global health organizations like FIGO and the International Confederation of Midwives (ICM) legitimized and reinforced these efforts and often helped open doors at regional and national levels.

LIBERALIZATION OF RESTRICTIVE LAWS AND POLICIES

Ipas Country Directors provided critical support to governments and many local groups (medical and human rights communities, parliamentarians, lawyers, women's organizations, community-based and youth organizations, and journalists) in their efforts to liberalize restrictive laws, policies, and practices. This has been a long and complex process in most countries. It has always been threatened by anti-abortion groups, including conservative members of the U.S. Congress and the "pro-life" lobby in the U.S., which has promoted and funded anti-abortion activities in countries around the world.

Some of the most dramatic examples of liberalization of restrictive abortion laws during the period I served as Ipas CEO are Nepal, Ethiopia, and Mexico City. In each of these cases, the Ipas Country Director and teams played a pivotal role, working with a variety of partners. They received valuable support and guidance from Charlotte Hord Smith, Ipas's Policy and Advocacy Director, and others, including Dr. Brookman-Amissah in Africa.

Nepal: In September 2002, the Nepalese Parliament voted to liberalize abortion as a way to promote safe motherhood and to ensure women's basic rights. This action followed years of advocacy for abortion law reform with the active engagement of civil society, the media, and Ministry of Health officials. All were concerned about the high levels of maternal mortality and morbidity from unsafe abortion. They were also alarmed by the number of women who were imprisoned for having an abortion while their rapists escaped charges.

In 2004, the Ministry of Health introduced the first comprehensive abortion care services at the Maternity Hospital in Kathmandu. Over the next few years, the Ministry expanded these services nationwide with the

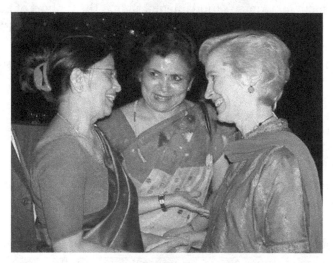

Talking to a senior Nepalese official (left) and Dr. Indira Basnett (center), 2008. MARY LUKE

support of Ipas and other organizations. Dr. Indira Basnett, Ipas Country Director, was pivotal in these major developments. By 2007, all districts of the country had at least one trained abortion provider. It was exciting to visit Nepal during this period and to witness the transformation underway in enabling women to obtain comprehensive abortion care.

In 2009, there was a landmark Supreme Court decision acknowledging that abortion was part of women's reproductive rights *and* human rights. Nepal is a great success story in helping women prevent and manage safely unwanted pregnancy although challenges remain to ensure access to safe abortion care in the country's tough terrain and under the limitations set by the U.S. as a major health donor.

Ethiopia: Beginning in 2002, Ipas was active in the process to revise the Ethiopian penal code to broaden the indications for abortion and worked with parliamentarians, members of civil society, and professional networks, including medical and women's groups. Following public debate and deliberations, the Parliament ratified in July 2004 a new clause in their penal code, allowing abortion in cases of rape, incest, risk to the life or health of the woman, fetal abnormality, when women are physically or mentally disabled, and in cases of minors who are physically or psychologically unprepared to raise a child.

Ipas assisted the Ministry of Health in drafting guidelines to implement the new law along with training health care providers and supporting the expansion of services throughout the country. This was done with the active engagement and brilliant leadership of Saba Kidanemariam, Ipas Country Director, and her team, collaborating with a network of committed individuals and organizations. Ethiopia is another example of impressive progress in a short period of time.

On one of my trips to Addis Ababa, I met with the president of Ethiopia (His Excellency Mr. Girma Wolde-Giorgis) to congratulate him and his government on the advances in reducing needless deaths and injuries due to unsafe abortion and increasing women's access to reproductive health information and services. I commented that Ethiopia served as a model for Africa in terms of high-level government commitment and action to improve the health and welfare of women and their families.

Both because of progress in addressing unsafe abortion and its overall

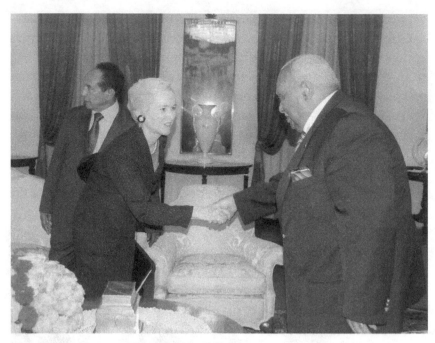

My meeting with the Ethiopian president, 2009. IPAS

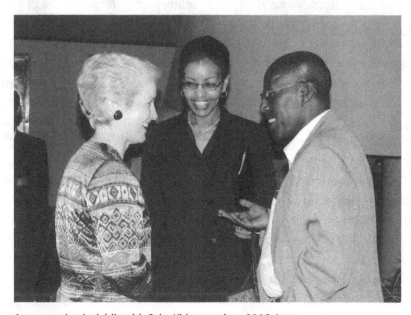

At a reception in Addis with Saba Kidanemariam, 2009. IPAS

role as a regional center in Africa, Ethiopia has served since 2003 as a site for several high-impact regional conferences on abortion organized by Ipas with other partners.

Mexico City: There was also an exciting development in Mexico City in April 2007 when the legislature decriminalized elective abortion in the first trimester of pregnancy and voted to make Ministry of Health facilities' services free of charge for residents in the Federal District; residents outside of Mexico City could receive services for a fee. At the same time, the law called for strengthening sex education in schools and ensuring widespread availability of contraceptives.

Ipas Mexico, under the leadership of Dr. Raffaela Schiavon, worked closely with the other member organizations of the Alianza Nacional por el Derecho a Decidir (National Alliance for the Right to Decide) to provide critical support to the government. They helped to develop and introduce new guidelines, train health care providers, and ensure access to appropriate technologies.

I was impressed during a visit to Mexico City in 2008 to see billboards and posters in many places, including in the metro system, advertising the new liberal abortion law and a popular hotline offering information on where to get legal abortion services at major hospitals in the Federal District. Following the law change, the use of MA skyrocketed from 25% of all legal abortions in 2007 to 83% seven years later. The actions taken in Mexico City provided a huge morale boost for other advocates in the Latin America region where there were still very restrictive laws on the books.

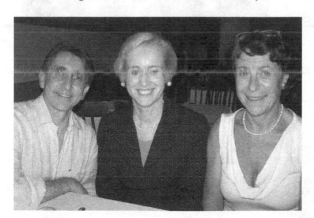

Discussing Ipas's partnership with the Secretaría de Salud in Mexico City, 2008: Dr. Patricio Sanhueza, Liz Maguire, and Dr. Raffaela Schiavon (left to right). MARY LUKE

Fortunately, the efforts of anti-abortion groups to challenge the easing of abortion restrictions were unsuccessful. The Mexican Supreme Court voted in August 2008 to uphold the new law.

India: The Medical Termination of Pregnancy (MTP) Act was passed in 1971, allowing termination of an unwanted pregnancy up to 20 weeks of gestation. Since 2006, Ipas (and subsequently the Ipas Development Foundation), under the leadership of Vinoj Manning, has been at the forefront of working with the government, FOGSI, and other civil society stakeholders to bring about a wider range of changes to the abortion law. This includes making first trimester abortion a woman's right, increasing the upper gestation limit for a variety of conditions, and most importantly, expanding the provider base to include nurses and midwives. These changes are critical to address the huge unmet need for comprehensive abortion care, especially in rural areas where there is a serious shortage of qualified health professionals. Ipas Development Foundation has helped the government with technical assistance, convening experts,

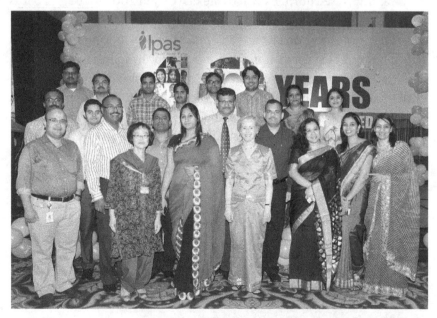

Celebrating Ipas's 40th anniversary with Ipas Development Foundation staff in Delhi, 2013: Vinoj Manning and Mary Luke (far left) and Liz Maguire (center). © IPAS DEVELOPMENT FOUNDATION (IDF)

and collating relevant evidence and global experience during the drafting of new amendments to the law and various consultations.

In March 2020, the Lok Sabha, the lower house of India's bicameral Parliament, approved limited amendments to the MTP Act. As of July 2020, the bill was awaiting approval of the upper house of the Parliament (Rajya Sabha) before becoming law. However, the current bill still does not go far enough in eliminating all barriers to women's access to safe abortion care. Sustained advocacy and more changes to the MTP Act will be needed.

During my tenure, Ipas provided funding for innovative initiatives in other countries in each region that resulted in the lifting of a range of restrictions on abortion-related care and improved guidelines. In South Africa, for example, the Choice on Termination of Pregnancy Act was amended in 2004 to enable registered midwives and nurses to provide abortion services. Ipas local staff were influential in facilitating this important change that greatly expanded women's access to quality care.

Other Ipas-supported countries where at least some progress was made in liberalizing restrictive laws or policies included, among others, Bangladesh, Bolivia, Brazil, Uruguay, Ghana, Kenya, Malawi, Mauritius, Mozambique, Nigeria, Swaziland, Zambia, and several Francophone African countries. We also focused on promoting liberal interpretation and full implementation of existing laws and policies as well as ensuring that post-abortion care and contraceptive information and services were available and accessible. Ipas staff celebrated every hard-fought policy advance and were poised to counter the challenges that inevitably occurred from the fierce anti-choice opposition. In the face of setbacks, we always redoubled our efforts.

ACCELERATING CHANGE IN REGIONAL AND GLOBAL FORA

Ipas was able to bring policy and programmatic advances in women's sexual and reproductive health and rights at the country level into discussions in regional and global fora and vice versa. Ensuring widespread dissemination of advances and sustained advocacy at every level proved to be a particularly effective strategy. We accomplished this by working with many different strategic partners and by supporting a wide range of activities. Through all these policy and advocacy initiatives, Barbara Crane, Charlotte Hord Smith, Dr. Eunice Brookman-Amissah, Leila Hessini, Kirsten Sherk (Public Affairs), and others were pivotal players, along with their teams, working with Ipas Country Directors and partner organizations.

Wherever reproductive health was on the agenda of regional and global conferences, Ipas advocated for the inclusion of issues related to maternal mortality and morbidity due to unsafe abortion and women's right to access contraception and comprehensive abortion care to reduce unwanted pregnancy. In partnership with other organizations, we elevated these issues by supporting conference participants, organizing sessions and pre-conference workshops on abortion, and delivering keynote addresses, papers, and statements. We also hosted side events, receptions, and press conferences, ensuring broad media coverage.

Ipas worked to mainstream abortion care in the medical community through strong support of the implementation of WHO guidelines on safe abortion along with participation in national and regional conferences as well as in every triennial Congress of FIGO and ICM. Ipas also actively supported the FIGO Working Group on Unsafe Abortion and its Consequences, led by Dr. Anibal Faundes.

We helped to influence language on reproductive health and safe abortion in UN Conferences following up on the 1994 International Conference on Population and Development in Cairo as well as the 1995 Fourth World Conference on Women in Beijing. Ipas was successful in building support to address abortion within UN treaty monitoring bodies and regional human rights law. We led sessions and side events on abortion at other major recurring global events such as the World Health Assembly, the Women Deliver Conference, the International Conference on Family Planning, the Association for Women's Rights in Development, and conferences on HIV/AIDS and sexual violence.

Regional conferences: Dr. Eunice Brookman-Amissah and the Ipas Africa Alliance for Women's Reproductive Health and Rights organized many workshops on unsafe abortion and participated in key conferences in the region reaching important constituencies. Through Dr. Brookman-Amissah's engagement with officials at the African Union (AU), there was a big breakthrough when African health ministers met in Maputo (under the auspices of the AU) in 2007 and committed to increasing access to safe abortion to the full extent of the law as part of the landmark Maputo Plan of Action.

In 2010, there was another historic regional conference, co-hosted by Ipas, in Ghana entitled Keeping our Promise: Eliminating Death and Injury from Unsafe Abortion in Africa. More than 230 participants from 24 countries shared experiences and developed new strategies to reduce unsafe abortion and increase access to contraception and safe abortion. Professor Fred Sai led the clarion call for action. In 2014, the African Commission on Human and Peoples' Rights issued a General Comment on access to safe abortion in the region, a major advance that was facilitated by Ipas efforts. Africa became the only world region to formally establish a human right to abortion.

During the period 2000–2015, Ipas played a pivotal role in similar reproductive health conferences and networks in Asia and Latin America, providing technical leadership and advocacy on abortion. One example of Ipas's influence was our engagement with the Latin American Consortium against Unsafe Abortion (CLACAI) aimed at supporting law reform and increased access to safe abortion. Through articles, workshops, and conferences, Ipas highlighted issues of sexual violence, unwanted pregnancy, and women's human rights designed to advance policy dialogue and change of restrictive laws and policies.

Global conferences: There were two historic global conferences organized and co-hosted by Ipas. The first Global Safe Abortion Conference was held in London in October 2007, with close to 800 participants from over 60 countries. Ipas partnered with Marie Stopes International in organizing this event. Our esteemed colleague Professor Fred Sai served as Chair.

In my opening remarks, I commented that:

This conference must mark a turning point for women's reproductive choices . . . . Together we must create the foundation for a new global movement to turn women's right to safe abortion into a reality . . . . When we share our Call to Action, we must say to everyone:

- *We will not stand for playing politics with women's lives.*

- *We will not allow powerful institutions to continue holding women and their defenders hostage on the issue of abortion.*

- *We will not stop until the basic technologies for safe abortion care and contraception, that have been available in rich countries for decades, reach every village in low-income countries around the world.*

- *We will not be satisfied until all women know their legal rights and reproductive options.*

- *We will not be silent until criminal penalties are removed for women who seek and health professionals who provide abortions.*

- *We will not rest until governments and donors put women's lives first in their priorities for money and attention.*

- *Most importantly, we will engage women everywhere to demand the sexual and reproductive health care they need and the compassionate treatment and respect they deserve . . . so that all women can prevent and mange unwanted pregnancies.*

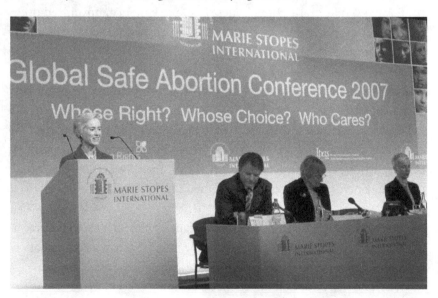

Speaking at the Global Safe Abortion Conference in London, 2007. IPAS

- *... Now is the time for all of us to speak out loudly and to take bold action. We must join together to stop the deaths and injuries from unsafe abortion, end the silence and hypocrisy, give voice to the voiceless, erase the stigma, and fight for social justice and equality, health and well-being for all women.*

During the plenary and breakout sessions, participants shared best practices in advocacy and service delivery and discussed the need to build and expand networks and coalitions in support of safe abortion care. The outcome of the conference was a strong Global Call to Action.

The second groundbreaking global event that Ipas co-hosted was the Conference on Uniting for Safe Legal Abortion, held in Airlie, Virginia in March 2014. Designed to be a much smaller event, conference participants included 60 leading advocates from 30 countries around the world. As Ipas CEO, I was a co-convener of the conference, along with Dr. Nafis Sadik (former Executive Director of UNFPA), Dr. Musimbi Kanyoro (President and CEO of the Global Fund for Women), and Ivens Reis Reyner (Youth Coalition for Sexual and Reproductive Rights in Brazil). Along with Ipas, co-sponsors of the conference were IPPF and the Center for Reproductive Rights. This conference was held two decades after the landmark ICPD in Cairo. In the interim 20 years, as I noted in my opening remarks, over one million women had died and more than 100 million women had suffered injuries from unsafe abortion, a wholly preventable cause.

We were all touched by the presence of Dr. Nafis Sadik who, in her mid-80s, spoke passionately about these issues and went on to highlight the importance of access to safe abortion in her remarks at the ICPD+20 meetings in April in New York. The *Airlie Declaration on Safe Legal Abortion* echoed many of the themes addressed in the first Global Safe Abortion Conference but went even farther. It called on governments and policymakers to:

... repeal laws that criminalize abortion and remove barriers on women's and girls' access to safe abortion services; release all women and girls and health care professionals who are incarcerated as a result of punitive abortion laws; make safe, legal abortion universally available, accessible and affordable for all women and girls; and invest

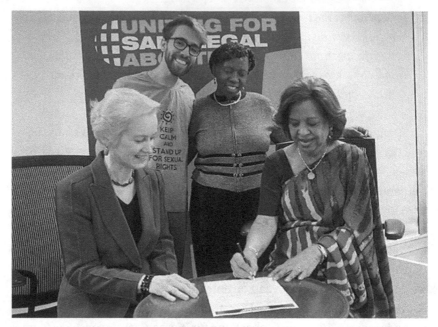

Signing the Airlie Declaration with Nafis Sadik (across from me) and Ivens Reis Reyner and Musimbi Kanyoro (behind us), 2014. IPAS

in effective preventive measures including comprehensive sexuality education, elimination of gender discrimination and sexual violence, and full access to all modern contraceptive methods . . . .

This was followed by a full-page ad in *The New York Times*, signed by conference participants, with a simple message: *Abortion is not a crime. It's a right . . . It should be safe, accessible, and legal for all women, everywhere.*

At the end of the conference, we held briefings on Capitol Hill and a press conference calling on the U.S. government to end permanently the Global Gag Rule that bans funding of abortion in its foreign aid program.

Empowering Advocates and Engaging the Media

Another dimension of Ipas's efforts to improve the policy environment was conducting a range of advocacy activities, including strategic use of the media. This work encompassed developing practical guides for advocates; a booklet entitled *Ten Facts about Abortion*, containing evidence-based responses to counter arguments of the anti-choice opposition; organizing national and regional meetings of advocacy groups; providing small grants to NGOs for support of their advocacy work; and promoting south-to-south exchanges on strategies and lessons learned. In addition, we trained journalists to ensure accurate reporting on sexual and reproductive health and rights, and organized press conferences and press releases for media outlets as well as gave frequent interviews to print and broadcast journalists. The annual September 28 Campaign for De-criminalization of Abortion was another effective vehicle for expanding advocacy work in Central and South America, and later globally.

Ipas shared the compelling stories of real women and girls in each region who underwent tremendous ordeals to terminate safely an unwanted pregnancy, often the result of rape or incest. These events happened in settings where abortion was highly restricted. Two of the stories were developed into documentary films that received widespread dissemination and use in multiple fora. One was *Rosita*, the story of a nine-year-old Nicaraguan girl who was raped and became pregnant and finally received, after considerable anguish, a safe abortion. The other film was entitled *Not Yet Rain: A Journey for Reproductive Freedom in Ethiopia*, produced by the Emmy Award-winner filmmaker Lisa Russell in association with Ipas. The film describes, in a powerful way, the stories of two young women dealing with an unwanted pregnancy and the difference that having a safe, legal abortion can make in the lives of women and their families. We showed this film to audiences in several cities in the U.S., including at a press briefing at the National Press Club in Washington, D.C.

Other materials Ipas published had a broad impact as well, including a report in 2013 entitled *When Abortion is a Crime: The Threat to Vulnerable Women in Latin America; Five Portraits: How safe abortion saves women's lives;* and *What can men do to support reproductive choice?*

LOBBYING TO EASE U.S. GOVERNMENT POLICY RESTRICTIONS

As an international NGO, Ipas's work was focused in developing countries, apart from more limited activities, as mentioned earlier, in the U.S. and Europe. These activities primarily involved training providers and ensuring availability of MVA. In addition, there was an innovative initiative entitled "MappingOurRights," under Leila Hessini, which addressed the sexual and reproductive rights of women of color, working with Sister-Song and other groups in the U.S. Ipas's most visible role in this country was lobbying on issues related to U.S. government restrictions on support for safe abortion overseas.

The Global Gag Rule (GGR): During my tenure as CEO, Ipas was a lead player, in partnership with several other organizations, in examining the negative impact of the Global Gag Rule. We assessed its effect on increasing unintended pregnancies, unsafe abortions, and maternal deaths and disabilities in developing countries. Early in the George W. Bush Administration, Ipas partnered with Population Action International and Planned Parenthood Federation of America on the Global Gag Rule Impact Project, which published a report entitled *Access Denied: U.S. Restrictions on International Family Planning*. The report provided evidence from several country programs supported by EngenderHealth and Pathfinder International. This was the first of many initiatives by Ipas and other organizations to document the adverse effect of the Global Gag Rule on the lives and health of women and their families around the world. The GGR has resulted in the disruption of vital family planning and other maternal and child health services and commodities, including HIV/AIDS prevention. Some of our Ipas Country Directors and staff participated in briefings on the Global Gag Rule with Bush Administration officials as well as with representatives and their staff on Capitol Hill.

A recent study conducted by Stanford University, published in *The Lancet*, covering the period 1995–2014, found that the Global Gag Rule increased abortion rates in sub-Saharan Africa by 40% as a result of the reduced ability of family planning organizations to provide modern contraceptives.

The Helms Amendment: At the beginning of the Obama Administration, we developed another major advocacy initiative, overseen by Barbara Crane, with the active engagement of Jamila Taylor, Patty Skuster, and others. Ipas created and chaired a Working Group on Helms Interpretation, which we convened regularly with other key partner organizations to lobby the Obama Administration to implement correctly the Helms Amendment to the U.S. Foreign Assistance Act. This action would allow for U.S. government support for the provision of abortion information and services for women in developing countries, where abortion is not being used "as a method of family planning" (i.e. rape, incest, and endangerment of the woman's life), where permitted by local law.

implications of US funding

On a trip to Ethiopia in November 2013, I saw yet another powerful example of how the Helms Amendment was denying access to safe abortion care even for women who are raped in a country where this service is legally allowed. If an Ethiopian woman lives near a public health facility that does not receive U.S. government funds, she can readily access a safe abortion, including counselling and contraception, in accordance with local law. However, for another Ethiopian woman whose nearest clinic is supported by USAID, the only service she can easily access if she wants to terminate an unwanted pregnancy is under the umbrella of sanctioned post-abortion care. This care is offered *after* the woman is already suffering or dying from a botched abortion.

I became so incensed by the injustice of this situation that I wrote a blog entitled "Two Women, Different Outcomes: How U.S. Foreign Assistance Policy Harms Women" published in *RH Reality Check* and *allAfrica*. In the blog, I profiled the cases of these Ethiopian women who were subjected to different treatment as a result of USAID funding. I asked the question, "How is it possible that U.S. foreign aid, which does so much good around the world, can also prevent a woman from receiving an abortion that is legal in her own country? The answer is overly restrictive interpretation of the Helms Amendment to the U.S. Foreign Assistance Act." The simple act of interpreting the Helms Amendment correctly, I wrote, "would enable millions of women, like Wubalem [in Ethiopia], to gain access to safe abortion care that is legal in their own country. It would no longer deny the rights of women in other countries to make their own reproductive choices freely and safely. Failure to act perpetuates an unconscionable imposition of U.S. abortion politics on women in developing countries who are least able to advocate for their own needs."

I had the privilege of working on the Helms Interpretation initiative with my committed Ipas colleagues as well as with a remarkable group of CEOs of other NGOs in the SRHR field. Those who were most active included Cecile Richards of Planned Parenthood Federation of America, Nancy Northup of the Center for Reproductive Rights, Suzanne Ehlers of Population Action International, Serra Sippel of the Center for Health and Gender Equity, Karl Hofmann of Population Services International, Pam Barnes of EngenderHealth, Ann Starrs of the Guttmacher Institute, and Purnima Mane of Pathfinder International, among others. We had several meetings with the highest-ranking members of the Obama White House to urge them to develop guidelines to implement fully the Helms Amendment. We also mobilized a broad coalition of partners and leaders from across the country who signed petitions to the White House on this issue.

Unfortunately, despite our persistent efforts, the Obama White House ultimately buckled under pressure from the Catholic Church and other religious organizations. This was an extremely disappointing development. What we were asking for was well within the limits of the law but had never been implemented since the Helms Amendment went into effect in 1973.

10

Building and Communicating the Evidence

Research, Monitoring, and Evaluation

During my tenure at Ipas, Janie Benson and her outstanding team developed a robust program of research, monitoring, and evaluation. Together, they produced safe abortion care indicators and designed, implemented, and evaluated studies on a wide range of issues. The research covered the availability and quality of comprehensive abortion care; the magnitude of unsafe abortion in Cambodia, Ethiopia, Kenya, Malawi, and Sierra Leone; and the costs of treating unsafe abortion. They also studied the performance of Ipas-trained clinicians as well as health care facilities we supported, providers' and women's experiences, and abortion stigma. In addition, they conducted a series of operations research studies to assess new service delivery approaches. All these studies represented a significant contribution to the international reproductive health field and had important policy and programmatic implications. One study showed, for example, that a shift from post-abortion care in Nigeria to safe legal abortion could reduce health system costs by 58%.

Ipas played a key role in assembling and sharing the latest advances through presentations at conferences as well as publications and articles in the peer-reviewed literature, posted on the website. There were many seminal articles written by Ipas staff during the period I was CEO. This long list includes one entitled "Unsafe abortion: the preventable pandemic," co-authored by David Grimes, Janie Benson, Susheela Singh, Bela Ganatra, and others and published in *The Lancet* in 2006. Another is "Counting Abortions so that Abortion Counts: Indicators for Monitoring the Availability and Use of Abortion Care Services," co-authored by Joan Healy, Karen Otsea, and Janie Benson and published in the *International Journal of Gynecology & Obstetrics* (2006).

Ipas was a co-founder of the Consortium for Research on Unsafe Abortion in Africa. This important body, which included Guttmacher Institute, the African Population and Health Research Center and other African-based organizations, collaborated on research, built research capacity in the region, and disseminated findings and recommendations of studies that promoted changes in abortion policies and programs. One of many noteworthy events was an African Regional Consultation on Linking Research to Action to End Unsafe Abortion in Sub-Saharan Africa, organized by Ipas and Consortium partners. Held in Addis in March 2006, the meeting was attended by over 120 researchers, policymakers, advocates, health care providers, and journalists from 13 African countries as well as representatives from international organizations and donors.

Along with the important studies conducted, the Ipas research and evaluation team continued to strengthen the organization's internal monitoring and evaluation systems and processes. This provided ready access to data on the number of women served by clinical trainees and Ipas-supported facilities, among other indicators. The latest systems ensured timely tracking and reporting of results, which were then shared with staff and donors. The data were made available through global dashboards, facilitating comprehensive analyses and recommendations for program improvements. During my country visits, I saw how these upgraded systems empowered our local staff and improved programs.

KNOWLEDGE SERVICES AND INFORMATION TECHNOLOGY

The essential organizational function of Knowledge Services and Information Technology (KSIT) was overseen during most of my time at Ipas by Eric Jones, working with a talented team. The Knowledge Services unit provided Ipas staff with the tools and services they needed to ensure that their work was evidence based and that they had easy access to a broad array of information essential to the performance of their specific duties. The Information Technology (IT) team managed a series of major upgrades to the organization's IT systems while I was CEO as well as provided ongoing training and support for staff at headquarters and in each of our country offices.

Ipas's Resource Center underwent an impressive evolution during my tenure. When I arrived in September 1999, Ipas's library consisted of a stack of boxes of books and papers. Under the direction of Julia Cleaver, the Ipas Resource Center became a premier global source of information on women's sexual and reproductive health and rights and comprehensive abortion care. These resources were used by staff, partners, and researchers around the world. The Ipas library was considered a knowledge leader in our field. In addition to all the Ipas publications and contributions to the peer-reviewed literature, it housed the extensive collection of Dr. Henry David, a well-known American psychologist and prodigious writer on contraception and abortion. We also developed *Ipas University* (*IpasU*), an online resource in English and Spanish for clinicians and others, with materials covering a variety of topics related to comprehensive abortion care as well as gender, sexual violence, values clarification, and human rights.

Thanks to the dedication, organizational skills, and hard work of Sally Fri, there is now an Ipas Archive at Duke University as part of a collaborative effort with the Sallie Bingham Center for Women's History and Culture and the Human Rights Archive. The David M. Rubenstein Rare Book & Manuscript Library is preserving the historical records, documents, and publications of Ipas for use by interested colleagues, students, and scholars.

COMMUNICATING IPAS'S MISSION AND WORK

Another critical area of work was evolving Ipas's communications strategies and programs under Marty Jarrell, Jennifer Daw Holloway, and their staff as well as Kirsten Sherk, head of Media Relations and Public Affairs. Anu Kumar was actively engaged in these activities and provided valuable guidance. In addition to developing and updating the website, one of the exciting activities was evolving periodically Ipas's logo, tagline, and key messages. The latest iteration of the logo was launched in January 2013 to mark Ipas's 40th anniversary. The new logo featured a symbol of a woman; the tagline highlighted the centrality of health, access, and rights. We wanted to convey the importance of reproductive health (including contraception and safe abortion) for women and girls along with enabling them to have ready access to high-quality information and services and to realize their sexual and reproductive rights.

The communications staff also produced several periodic publications and e-newsletters. Together with colleagues from across the organization, they made extensive use of print, broadcast, and rapidly evolving social media and other networks to report on Ipas's work. All these initiatives, along with the advocacy activities described earlier, expanded Ipas's voice, presence, and impact around the world and highlighted the importance of women being able to control their reproductive lives and their futures.

11

RESPONSIBILITIES, CHALLENGES, AND OPPORTUNITIES AS CEO

Serving as CEO of a global non-profit brings major responsibilities as well as many opportunities, rewards, and challenges. I was privileged to work with a dedicated, cross-cultural, multi-disciplinary, and multi-generational team. Like every CEO of an international non-profit, I reported to the Board of Directors and had overall responsibility for preserving the mission, vision, and values of the organization; developing and overseeing the implementation of the latest strategic plan and annual budget; fundraising; and ensuring strong fiscal, programmatic, and management oversight as well as operational effectiveness. I also focused on maintaining excellent communications with the Board and staff; creating and sustaining an open and supportive work environment; working effectively with partners; and representing the organization before many different constituencies, including the media.

Carrying out all these responsibilities was a constant juggling act, but one on which I thrived. It required continual scanning of the external and internal environment and strong planning and management skills along with the ability to work on many different activities at the same time. I had to respond promptly and effectively to changing circumstances and make whatever adjustments were needed along the way, while generally maintaining a calm demeanor and grounded optimism.

Like every CEO, I had some memorable and challenging experiences. Early in my tenure, there was a moment of high anxiety when a colleague

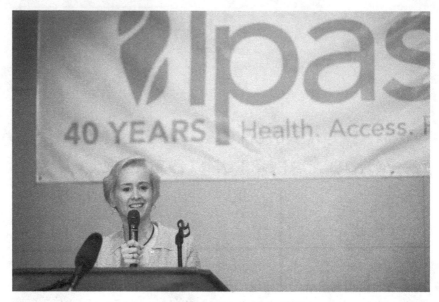

Speaking at an event celebrating Ipas's 40th anniversary, 2013. IPAS

and I got lost and showed up late for an appointment with Ipas's major donor. We feared we might lose funding that was essential for the organization's work. Fortunately, we received a warm welcome and had a successful meeting. Another memorable moment happened in Mexico City where I was visiting our Ipas team and partners. I was asked to give a speech in Spanish at a special event for senior officials. In the middle of my remarks, the power went out and the room became dark. It was impossible to read my notes. What followed was, in my mind, a prolonged interruption. To my great relief, the blackout lasted only a couple of minutes, and I was able to finish my speech without too much awkwardness. These are just two examples of some embarrassing moments.

There were a few times during my 16 years as president when I regretted a remark or decision I made. Most challenges concerned issues related to different aspects of Ipas's international work, operations, personnel, or funding. Overall, I loved serving as CEO of Ipas. The job was enormously energizing and fulfilling. I was excited to work each day on a critical mission with such committed and accomplished colleagues.

Along with my daily responsibilities at Ipas, I enjoyed interacting regularly with CEOs of other international reproductive health and rights organizations and attending the semi-annual meetings where we discussed important issues facing our field and common concerns. There were many opportunities during my tenure to speak at international, regional, and national conferences in every region. I participated in numerous press conferences and authored or co-authored articles, reports, and blogs. Another stimulating and rewarding experience was serving as a Board member of several sister organizations in the SRHR field. This included six years as a trustee of the Population Reference Bureau in Washington, D.C. and a similar tenure as a founding Board member and Co-Chair of the Safe Abortion Action Fund headquartered in London. In addition, I was Board Chair of WomanCare Global International for four years.

Enhancing Organizational Efficiency and Effectiveness

From our headquarters in Chapel Hill, I focused on building Ipas's technical, programmatic, and policy leadership and expanding the organization's funding base. Another high priority was strengthening finance and administration and general operations. To increase Ipas's overall effectiveness and efficiency, we prioritized organizational development and conducted several restructuring exercises during my tenure to ensure alignment with new strategic plans and programs. We continued to decentralize operations and upgrade our human and financial resource functions along with our global communications and support to staff. There were many capacity-building workshops as well as professional development opportunities. We also implemented measures to ensure the safety and security of staff, especially our overseas teams.

The powerful new information systems we developed were essential to support Ipas's expanded work and field presence. All these measures entailed substantial time, effort, and resources, as did dealing with staff-related issues. Most importantly, in response to problems in a couple of country offices where we discovered weak management and insufficient financial controls, we built and implemented a comprehensive financial compliance plan, hired a Chief Compliance Officer (Michael Shawkey) and strengthened risk management and accountability. Every large international organization encounters these kinds of issues and must take prompt, appropriate action as well as ensure effective monitoring and oversight along with continuous capacity building.

In general, whenever faced with serious problems, I tried to look at them as opportunities for improvement. Some challenges were bigger than others, but none were insurmountable, especially working as a team committed to finding the best solutions.

SUPPORTING AND EMPOWERING THE STAFF

A high priority was to inspire personal and professional excellence among the staff, provide daily encouragement and positive feedback, and maintain Ipas's family-oriented environment. We worked extremely hard as a team but always took time to have fun. We had regular birthday parties and other staff celebrations. We also hosted an annual Halloween party that showcased the many other talents of staff who took on different personalities and performed brilliant skits. Once a year, I became Martine Lambeau, my imaginary redheaded French friend who ran a reproductive health clinic in Nice. She wore a sparkling, tight-fitting outfit and spoke

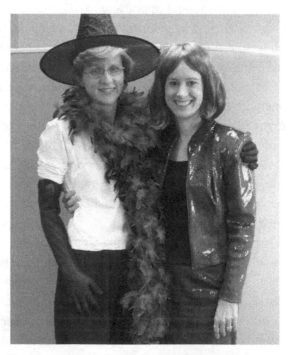

Ann Leonard and "Martine," 2009. IPAS

heavily accented English. On these and other occasions, my colleagues and I laughed a lot and enjoyed a welcomed break from work.

We also celebrated Thanksgiving together, and everyone contributed a dish to the abundant annual pre-Thanksgiving feast at the office in Chapel Hill. This was an opportunity for me to thank staff and to recognize those who had reached milestone work anniversaries. I made sure that Country Directors had similar opportunities to host parties for their staff. I strongly supported Ipas staff having a balance between home life and work and was always impressed with how colleagues helped each other in times of personal hardship and loss. Among the events I enjoyed the most were the lunches I had with each Ipas unit in Chapel Hill where I could hear first-hand, in an informal setting, about everyone's work, ask and answer questions, and reiterate my thanks for their commitment and hard work.

The most celebratory occasions were when the Country Directors came to Chapel Hill and we honored these exceptional leaders at parties and special events, including fashion shows. There was always a lot of laughter, music, and dancing. When the Country Directors got together, they would discuss their policy and programmatic initiatives, what was working well and what was not, their challenges, lessons learned, bold new ideas, and recommendations. I was inspired by the camaraderie among them and with staff across the organization.

Ipas was indeed fortunate to have many of the best and brightest in the sexual and reproductive health and rights field around the world,

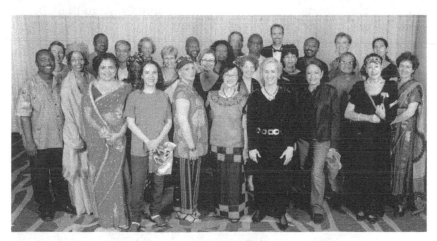

Ipas Country Directors and other senior staff, 2011. IPAS

including a growing number of young people with creative ideas and lots of enthusiasm. It was rewarding to see them take on increasing levels of responsibility and do a terrific job. We had some wonderful support staff, too. Bettie Seymour was the Ipas receptionist and the warm and welcoming voice of the Chapel Hill office—on the phone and in person. Bettie and I had a tradition of exchanging "bear hugs" at least once a week.

GOVERNANCE AND BOARD EVOLUTION

Another dynamic area was ensuring strong working relationships with the Board as it continued to evolve during my tenure. As CEO and an ex-officio Board member, I worked with the Chair and members of the Executive Committee and other committee chairs on improving the composition and functioning of the Board as they carried out their governance, legal, fiduciary, audit, risk management, and other responsibilities in accordance with the bylaws. Together, we dealt with any major issues, strengthened operations, and built a diverse, more prominent international Board.

In addition to Professor Fathalla of Egypt, the Ipas Board included over the years other great pioneers in the field of women's reproductive health and rights such as Jemima Dennis-Antwi of Ghana; Angela Kamara of Liberia; the Honorable Njoki Ndungu of Kenya; Grace Delano, Bene Madunagu, and Dr. Otobo Ujah of Nigeria; Dr. Eddie Mhlanga of South Africa; and Dr. Davy Chikamata of Zambia. We were also fortunate to have Amulya Ratna Nanda and Dr. Nozer Sheriar of India, Arzu Rana Deuba of Nepal (Member of Parliament and wife of the former Prime Minister), Ellen Hardy and Dr. Mabel Bianco of Argentina, Fred Nunes of Jamaica, Gabriela Cano and Dr. Rafael Lozano of Mexico, and Lilian Abracinskas of Uruguay. It was important to have several Europeans serve on the Board, too. We welcomed Dr. Hans Vemer and Dr. Paul Van Look of the Netherlands, Dr. Berit Austveg of Norway, Dr. Jerker Liljestrand of Sweden, and Dilys Cossey of the U.K., as well as Tracey Ramsay of Canada.

From the U.S, we had well-known experts in the SRHR field, such as Dr. Joe Speidel, Amy Tsui, Jane Bertrand, Marie Bass, Gordon Duncan, Mary Fjerstad, Geoffrey Knox, and Sheila Maher, among others. There were various prominent figures already on the Board when I joined. They included Dr. Pouru Bhiwandi, Dr. Paul Blumenthal, Lance Bronnenkant,

Nicki Gamble, Anne Firth Murray, Dr. Louise Tyrer, Dr. Don Minkler, and Jael Silliman. Lida Coleman, Deb DeWitt, and Lou Zellner, among others, brought extensive expertise to lead and staff the Finance and Audit Committees. Jolynn Dellinger provided a valuable legal perspective.

I am grateful for the guidance and support I received from the Board during my tenure and for the many special friendships. I am especially indebted to Pouru Bhiwandi for her pivotal role in bringing me to Ipas in 1999, for the close bond we developed, and for her long and dedicated service to the staff and Board of the organization, including her time as Board Chair.

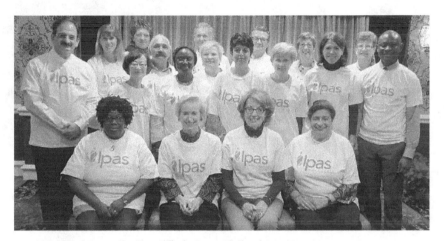

Ipas Board and Executive Team displaying new Ipas logo, 2013. Ipas

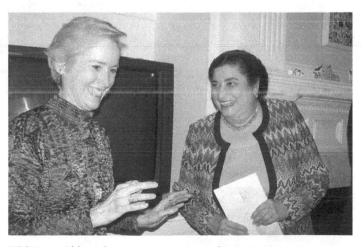

With Pouru Bhiwandi at an Ipas event at my house, 2010

12

Accomplishments
of the Ipas Team

Soon after I joined Ipas, I adopted the theme of "Accelerating the Pace of Change in support of Women's Reproductive Health and Rights around the world." With the extraordinary efforts of the Ipas staff, the contributions of the Board, and the engagement of many partners and donors, we were successful in accomplishing this goal. Ipas has served as a catalyst for change at every level—locally, nationally, regionally, and globally.

During my sixteen years, the organization's annual income increased seven-fold, from about $9 million to a high of $65 million, with a greatly expanded donor base. We also laid the foundation for an individual fundraising campaign after relying almost exclusively on grants from foundations and foreign governments. Over the same period, the staff size quintupled (from approximately 100 to nearly 500), with the overseas offices increasing from four to 15, along with activities in another 10 to 15 countries.

Buttressed by strong country offices and two regional offices, Ipas transformed into a large, global non-profit with an extensive network of government and non-governmental partners dedicated to reducing unsafe abortion and advancing women's sexual and reproductive health and rights. From 2000–2015, the collective work of Ipas and many other organizations had an important impact on saving and enhancing women's lives across the developing world, especially among the poor, young, and most vulnerable.

While remaining laser-focused on Ipas's unique mission, we succeeded in enhancing considerably the organization's visibility, reach, and impact by continual innovation and taking bold action. Ipas helped put the critical need for comprehensive abortion care, including family planning, on the global development agenda. Our staff organized trainings for tens of thousands of ob-gyns, mid-level providers, and other health care workers as well as helped support public and private health facilities. We distributed over 1.5 million MVA kits during my tenure, providing at least 40 million women with safe uterine evacuation. In addition, by working with a wide range of partners, we contributed to a dramatic increase in the number of women gaining access to medical abortion and contraception to prevent repeat unintended pregnancies.

Also notable, as discussed earlier, were the many changes during this period in restrictive laws, policies, and practices related to women's sexual and reproductive health and rights. Ipas played a key role in institutionalizing legal and policy improvements across more than 20 countries benefitting tens of millions of women. We also influenced the debate in regional and global arenas and helped moved the field from "safe abortion, where legal" to "safe, legal abortion everywhere," as a woman's fundamental human right.

It was gratifying to watch the evolution of country programs and their broad impact, especially the comprehensive and mature programs in countries such as Mexico, Bolivia, Brazil, Ghana, Ethiopia, Kenya, Nigeria, South Africa, Zambia, Bangladesh, India, Nepal, and Vietnam, among others. The program in India is one example of an important success story, led by Vinoj Manning and his outstanding staff. Starting in 2000 with small activities in three districts of one state, the program grew to a very large one, covering 12 states. It provided a wide range of services, supporting the Ministry of Health and Family Welfare at the national and state levels. In 2008, Ipas India was registered as a not-for-profit organization known as the Ipas Development Foundation (IDF) and has since been a vital partner of Ipas. IDF has been recognized for several years as one of the top 10 great mid-size workplaces in India, thanks to visionary and supportive leadership and a talented and empowered team.

Working in one of the world's most difficult political environments, Marta María Blandón, Ipas Director for Central America, was a brilliant

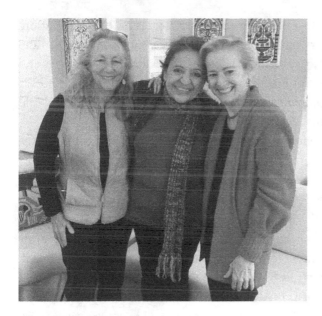

Appreciating time with special friends and former Ipas colleagues Virginia Chambers (left) and Marta María Blandón (center), 2018.
ALEJANDRA MACHADO

strategist and fearless champion of the reproductive health and rights of women and girls in the region. Along with fighting for the liberalization of highly restrictive abortion laws and the removal of punitive practices, the Ipas Central America team supported the training of health care providers and the expansion of women's access to contraception and post-abortion care.

I am equally proud of the huge contributions Ipas staff made in the area of technical innovations, especially the improvements in uterine evacuation and expanded contraceptive choice. Other major innovations included the updated training curricula, new standards and guidelines for service delivery, clinical guidance, and the widespread use of "values clarification." Ipas provided strong leadership in addressing the needs of adolescents and young adults and mobilizing community action, as well as tackling stigma and discrimination. The advances in monitoring, research and evaluation, and increased use of mass and social media are also impressive.

When I joined Ipas, I commented on what I felt were the organization's special characteristics: creative, collaborative, entrepreneurial, risk-taking, trailblazing, and mission driven. These attributes continued during my tenure. Ipas's successes were the result of an extraordinary team effort made up of passionate, talented leaders at all levels of the organization, including a group of dynamic young leaders. We pursued bold ideas and strategies, leveraged strategic partnerships for maximum impact, and persevered in the face of many political and sociocultural obstacles. We were committed to knowledge sharing, continuous learning, and organizational improvement.

Finally, I am indebted to the Board as well as all the donors—large and small—who believed in the mission, work, and staff of Ipas. They reported that they received good value for their investment. Throughout my 16 years, I welcomed each day with optimism and enthusiasm, even during challenging times. I remained dedicated to providing passionate and compassionate leadership, strong strategic direction, and a supportive enabling environment to fuel Ipas's growth, innovation, and impact. I often considered my role to be akin to that of an orchestra conductor, facilitating the work of a gifted staff and making sure that Ipas continued to fulfill its mandate, take courageous action, and work effectively with partners at all levels. Most importantly, we made a difference in the lives of the women and adolescents we served around the world.

PASSING THE BATON

My tenure at Ipas was immensely rewarding. This was due to the mission and the exceptional staff who shared part or all those years with me, along with the amazing people I met in every region. In mid-2014, I determined that it was time to pass the baton to a new generation of leaders. I gave the Board a year's notice before I retired the following summer. During my final year at Ipas, I had a chance to express, in writing and in person, my deep appreciation to Board and staff members, donors, the CEOs of partner organizations, and other friends and colleagues in the international reproductive health and rights community.

In June 2015, I was treated to two retirement parties, one in Chapel Hill and the other in Washington, D.C. At the Ipas Board meeting in Chapel Hill, I reiterated my gratitude to the directors, my Executive Team, and my front office staff and handed out small gifts of appreciation. At the big farewell party with the Chapel Hill-based staff the following evening, I was overwhelmed and humbled by all the tributes, including an album of photos of all the country teams who were unable to be there and a book of remembrances completed by Ipas staff which I will always treasure. I was also showered with gifts and commendations. It was a festive event and one I will never forget. I called on the staff to keep up the fight for women's basic human rights and repeated the call to action that I had made at the 2007 Global Safe Abortion Conference. At the end, I underscored that "Ipas's commitment to this agenda is unwavering. We are *undaunted* in the struggle for women's health, access, and rights!"

The reception held in Washington, D.C. at the end of June was also wonderful. The group included friends and colleagues from different stages of my career. It was exciting to talk to people whom I had not seen in quite a while, especially many of my USAID friends, and to chat with CEOs of partner organizations. My brother flew from California and Jane Bertrand from New Orleans to join the festivities, along with Terry from Chapel Hill, which made the evening truly special. I was touched by the thoughtful remembrances and pleased that I was able to convey my thanks to all those present. Following the reception, the current and former Chairs of the Ipas Board who served during my tenure graciously hosted a dinner in my honor that I deeply appreciated. We had several more hours to exchange memories and laughter.

In mid-July 2015, it was time to leave Ipas. I will remain forever grateful for this chapter of my career. While there have been significant changes in the organization since I retired, I am pleased that, under the strong leadership of Anu Kumar, Ipas is continuing to innovate and play an effective role in advancing women's sexual and reproductive health and rights around the world.

PART FOUR

REVIEWING THE UNFINISHED AGENDA

SEXUAL AND REPRODUCTIVE HEALTH AND RIGHTS FOR ALL

13

Progress to Date

In pursuing my mission of helping women around the world make their own reproductive choices freely and safely, I feel privileged to have worked for three unique institutions spanning more than four decades. The Population Reference Bureau, established in 1929, provides information to U.S. and overseas audiences about population, health, and the environment and "empowers people around the world to use this information to advance the well-being of current and future generations." USAID is the world's largest family planning and reproductive health donor providing comprehensive support to programs in every region. It has had a huge global impact over the past 55 years. And Ipas, created in 1973, is the only international non-governmental organization devoted exclusively to supporting women's access to comprehensive abortion care, including family planning, as well as championing their sexual and reproductive rights.

Twenty-five years after the historic 1994 International Conference on Population and Development (ICPD) in Cairo, the SRHR community has been assessing achievements to date and the road ahead. There have been a series of comprehensive reports and articles on these issues in the last few years. I appreciate the thorough analysis of the available evidence, and the findings and recommendations of *Our future: a Lancet commission on adolescent health and wellbeing (2016)*, *Abortion Worldwide 2017: Uneven Progress and Unequal Access* published by Guttmacher Institute, and the 2018 Guttmacher-*Lancet* Commission's report.*Accelerate progress—sexual and reproductive health and rights for all*. Other important reports include: UNFPA's *State of World Population 2020—Against My Will*, and its 2019 report—*Unfinished Business*, as well as *FP2020 Women at the*

Center 2018–2019: Media Coverage. In addition, there are the presentations, statements, and articles from the 2019 Nairobi Summit, including the background document commissioned by UNFPA entitled *Sexual and Reproductive Health and Rights: An Essential Element of Universal Health Coverage*, and *Accelerating the Promise: The Report on the Nairobi Summit on ICPD25.*

Since the approval of the 1994 ICPD Programme of Action, we witnessed significant advances in expanding women's and girls' access to contraception and reproductive health information and services in developing countries along with major declines in maternal mortality and morbidity. The improvements in a range of indicators reflect technological and programmatic innovations and the dedicated efforts and resources of individuals, governments, intergovernmental agencies, international and local NGOs, foundations, other generous donors, and the commercial sector. However, the progress in each region has been both uneven and inadequate, especially among poor and vulnerable populations.

CORE COMPONENTS OF SRHR

Family planning and reproductive health services are critical to the autonomy of women and girls and their overall well-being. Efforts over the past 25 years have been directed at: enabling women and girls to choose whether, when, and with whom to have children; reducing high-risk pregnancies and allowing sufficient spacing between pregnancies; decreasing unintended pregnancies and increasing access to safe abortion care and contraception; reducing deaths of mothers, children, and infants; helping to prevent new HIV infections and mother-to-child transmission; and decreasing harmful practices such as female genital mutilation. All these factors contributed to improved health, economic growth, and the reduction of poverty. However, this happened *before* COVID-19 hit.

In the area of family planning, UNFPA reports that use of modern contraception increased from 470 million to 840 million women between 1990 and 2018. The quality of care overall improved substantially as well, although there are considerable variations by geographic area. A 2019 report by the Center for Global Development underscored the many benefits of family planning, commenting that it is "central to advancing the multi-sectoral goals of individuals, communities, nations, and the planet."

The global maternal mortality ratio declined by about 44% in the same period. One reason for this drop is increased access to information and simple technologies for safe abortion care, resulting in fewer women and girls suffering and dying needlessly from unsafe abortion.

Since the Cairo Conference, there has also been significant progress in the prevention and treatment of sexually transmitted infections, including HIV/AIDS. In addition, the proportion of girls in countries where female genital mutilation is widely prevalent fell from 49% to 31%. However, UNFPA notes that the total number of women and girls impacted by harmful practices increased due to population growth.

There have been some advances in addressing other key issues, including respecting the human rights of lesbian, gay, bisexual, trans, queer, and other (LGBTQ+) people. But progress varies substantially by country and region. Prejudice, discrimination, and violence toward LGBTQ+ individuals remain a major problem, especially in the developing world.

14

Huge Unmet Needs

All individuals have a right to access sexual and reproductive health (SRH) information and services that are critical to leading healthy and fulfilling lives. These services must adhere to high medical standards and include quality counselling and respect for the right to privacy, confidentiality, and informed consent; they must be free of coercion, discrimination, and violence. Information about self-care and pills should also be available, especially in situations where medical services are inaccessible for various reasons, including during the latest global coronavirus pandemic.

Family Planning and Comprehensive Abortion Care

Despite the advances, the level of current unmet need for family planning and safe abortion care—as well as for other aspects of reproductive health, rights, and gender equality—is enormous. In 2017, over 214 million women of reproductive age in the developing world wanted to delay or avoid pregnancy but were not using a modern method of contraception, representing almost one out of every four women aged 15–49. For sexually active adolescents aged 15–19, the unmet need for contraception was 60%.

Failure to use contraception is due to a wide variety of reasons: limited access to contraceptive information and counselling; over-confidence about not getting pregnant; lack of informed consent or freedom to select the method that best meets an individual's needs; lack of spousal or partner support; and factually incorrect information. Other factors are high cost of care; poor quality of services; lack of confidentiality; provider bias;

fear of, or actual, side effects; inconvenience; contraceptive stock-outs; stigma and cultural opposition; as well as legal, policy, and other barriers.

Fortunately, there is a wide range of modern contraceptive methods, including a number that are 99% effective with correct and consistent use. However, many methods have high user discontinuation rates. Since no contraceptive is 100% effective or is used correctly and consistently 100% of the time, there will always be unintended or unwanted pregnancies and recourse to abortion.

A study published in July 2020 in *The Lancet Global Health* estimates that each year there are 121 million unintended pregnancies worldwide and 73.3 million (or 61%) ending in abortion. The sheer magnitude of abortions globally has been highlighted graphically by Dr. Nozer Sheriar, former Secretary General of FOGSI, when he said, "What would happen if all women who had an abortion over the last 10 years came together? They would form the world's third LARGEST country."

The 2018 Guttmacher-*Lancet* Commission report noted that 50% of abortions in developing countries are unsafe, reaching a high of 88% in middle Africa. Estimates at that time indicated that approximately 25 million women and girls annually undergo an unsafe abortion because they cannot access quality care. This happens because of restrictive laws, policies, and practices; insufficient information; stigma; cost; distance; unnecessary regulations; spousal or partner disapproval; and the refusal of trained practitioners to provide legal abortions; as well as other barriers.

No woman or girl should have to put her life or health at risk because she does not have access to the information and services she needs. According to WHO, abortion is an extremely simple, safe, and effective procedure when performed by a health care provider with the necessary skills, using appropriate technologies. These include vacuum aspiration and medical abortion (using a pharmaceutical regimen) which is a popular, non-invasive option and can be used by women in their own homes.

We know that outlawing or restricting abortion does not decrease the number of abortions; instead, it increases needless deaths and disabilities. Treating the serious complications of unsafe abortion is estimated at more than a half billion dollars a year. There would be practically zero deaths or disabilities if all women and girls received sexuality education, used an effective modern method of contraception, had ready access to safe, legal abortion, and obtained prompt care for the complications of unsafe abortion.

Although there has been progress in liberalizing laws, policies, and practices, abortion in many countries remains highly stigmatized as well as severely restricted; in some countries, it is enforced through criminal penalties on women and providers. Every day, women and girls are denied the care to which they are entitled as a matter of human rights. For all women and girls, abortion should be safe, legal, accessible, and affordable.

U.S. POLICY RESTRICTIONS IMPEDE ACCESS TO SRH SERVICES

U.S. government assistance to SRHR programs in Africa, Asia, and Latin America has been dramatically restricted by the expanded Global Gag Rule imposed by President Trump, resulting in an increase in unintended pregnancies and abortions.

In the U.S., in recent years, there has been an unprecedented attack on women's constitutionally protected right to safe abortion. This fundamental right is increasingly threatened given the current composition of the U.S. Supreme Court. Moreover, many states under Republican governors and legislatures have successfully closed clinics. Access to legal abortion has been severely limited through a range of tactics. These include intimidation by protesters at abortion clinics; provision of false or biased information; and burdensome requirements such as mandatory counselling, waiting periods, and parental consent. There are also medically unnecessary tests, onerous licensing standards for clinics, and stipulations that abortion providers must be affiliated with a local hospital. All these restrictions, plus the cost of services, result in delays and barriers for at least 40 million women of reproductive age in the U.S.

In July 2019, the Trump Administration imposed a ban on abortion referrals at U.S. family planning clinics supported by Title X government funds. An estimated 40% of Title X patients in the U.S. had been served by Planned Parenthood Federation of America (PPFA) facilities that care for millions of women every year. Following this punitive action, PPFA withdrew from Title X funding, leaving it with the major task of raising additional funds to try to cover some of the needs. The greatest impact is depriving poor and young women of ready access not only to safe abortion, but also to family planning, emergency contraception, and other important reproductive health services, including cancer screenings and the prevention and treatment of sexually transmitted infections.

OTHER CRITICAL NEEDS

There are huge unmet needs around the world in other aspects of sexual and reproductive health as well. According to the 2018 Guttmacher-*Lancet* Commission report, *each year* in the developing world: over 30 million women still give birth outside health facilities; over 45 million don't receive any, or at best inadequate, antenatal care; a minimum of 350 million men and women will need treatment for curable sexually transmitted infections; and close to two million people become newly infected with HIV. In addition, the number of women in developing countries suffering and dying from cervical cancer is unacceptably high when this is a largely preventable disease.

Other pressing unmet needs are ensuring that adolescents and women can receive comprehensive sexuality education and make voluntary and informed decisions about their sexual and reproductive health. Counselling and services for sexual health and well-being are also critical. Much remains to be done to address prevention and treatment of gender-based violence, another violation of human rights. It is devastating to know that one-third of all women have been coerced into sex, beaten, or abused!

Greater efforts are needed to increase coverage of essential maternal and newborn health as well as reduce high levels of infertility. There are also the massive tasks of eliminating child marriage and deaths from HIV/AIDS. Female genital mutilation affects over 200 million women and girls in 30 countries; this figure could rise by another 68 million because of population growth.

Moreover, there are distinct SRH needs among special populations who generally face increased obstacles, discrimination, and risks. In addition to young people, there are people with disabilities; individuals of diverse sexual orientations, gender identities, and sex characteristics; sex workers; drug users; racial and ethnic minorities; and migrants.

Another neglected but important area is addressing the SRH needs of men and boys. Furthermore, men and boys should be systematically involved as active supporters of women and girls making their own decisions regarding their bodies and rights, including gaining access to the information and services they need. Initiatives aimed at engaging men as partners have proven effective and must be greatly expanded.

Finally, there is the sobering reality that the gaps in coverage, range, and quality of SRH services are greatest among the urban and rural poor and less educated. This is also true for displaced and refugee populations, estimated to be over 70 million people in 2018 and growing each year.

It is important to underscore that the estimates provided in this chapter of the high unmet SRH needs *predate* the COVID-19 pandemic. Decades of social and economic progress could now be lost because of this global crisis.

15

THE CHALLENGES AHEAD

THE NAIROBI SUMMIT AND BEYOND

ICPD25 was held in the capital of Kenya, 12–14 November 2019. At the Nairobi Summit, there were over 8,300 participants from 172 countries and territories, representing national governments, international institutions, civil society, youth, and the private sector, among others. With UNFPA and the governments of Kenya and Denmark serving as co-conveners, the conference underscored the imperative to "intensify our efforts for the full, effective and accelerated implementation and funding of the ICPD Programme of Action . . . , the outcomes of its reviews, and Agenda 2030 for Sustainable Development."

During the conference and its 150 sessions, participants focused on the need to dramatically increase efforts in five major areas: achieving universal access to sexual and reproductive health and rights as part of universal health coverage (UHC); addressing sexual and gender-based violence and harmful practices; mobilizing the required financing to complete the ICPD Programme of Action and sustain the gains made; drawing on demographic diversity to drive economic growth and achieve sustainable development; and upholding the right to sexual and reproductive health services in humanitarian and fragile contexts.

The final *Nairobi Statement on ICPD25: Accelerating the Promise* includes specific commitments in each of these areas by 2030. The goals listed in the Statement include the following:

- *Zero unmet need for family planning information and services, and universal availability of quality, accessible, affordable and safe modern contraceptives.*

- *Zero preventable maternal deaths and maternal morbidities, such as obstetric fistulas, by, inter alia, integrating a comprehensive package of sexual and reproductive health interventions, including access to safe abortion to the full extent of the law, measures for preventing and avoiding unsafe abortions, and for the provision of post-abortion care, into national UHC strategies, policies and programmes, and to protect and ensure all individuals' right to bodily integrity, autonomy and reproductive rights, and to provide access to essential services in support of these rights.*

- *Access for all adolescents and youth, especially girls, to comprehensive and age-responsive information, education and adolescent-friendly comprehensive, quality and timely services to be able to make free and informed decisions and choices about their sexuality and reproductive lives, to adequately protect themselves from unintended pregnancies, all forms of sexual and gender-based violence and harmful practices, sexually transmitted infections, including HIV/AIDS, to facilitate a safe transition into adulthood.*

- *Zero sexual and gender-based violence and harmful practices, including zero child, early and forced marriage as well as zero female genital mutilation.*

- *Elimination of all forms of discrimination against all women and girls, in order to realize all individuals' full socio-economic potential.*

- *Investing in the education, employment opportunities, health, including family planning and sexual and reproductive health services, of adolescents and youth, especially girls, so as to fully harness the promises of the demographic dividend.*

- *Building peaceful, just and inclusive societies, where no one is left behind, where all, irrespective of race, colour, religion, sex, age, disability, language, ethnic origin, sexual orientation and gender identity or expression, feel valued, and are able to shape their own destiny and contribute to the prosperity of all societies.*

- *Committing to the notion that nothing about young people's health and well-being can be discussed and decided upon without their meaningful involvement and participation.*

- *Ensuring that the basic humanitarian needs and rights of affected populations, especially that of girls and women, are addressed as critical components of responses to humanitarian and environmental crises, as well as fragile and post-crisis reconstruction contexts, through the provision of access to comprehensive sexual and reproductive health information, education and services, including access to safe abortion services to the full extent of the law, and post-abortion care, to significantly reduce maternal mortality and morbidity, sexual and gender-based violence, and unplanned pregnancies under these conditions.*

These ambitious goals are all critical. The *Nairobi Statement* contains others that relate to mobilizing the required financing as well as data collection and use. However, the one area of SRHR that did not emerge from the conference with a bold goal was the elimination of unsafe abortion and the achievement of universal access to safe, *legal* abortion. Enabling all women and girls to exercise this fundamental human right is an essential step in achieving zero preventable maternal deaths and morbidities. This requires removing restrictive laws, policies, and practices around the world that impede women's access to safe abortion.

At the time of the Nairobi Summit, there was a counter-event with representatives from the U.S., Kenya, and several other countries protesting key elements of ICPD25, including abortion. The Trump Administration officials who attended the conference provided a dramatic contrast to the U.S. government's role at the 1994 ICPD in Cairo where the U.S. delegation was a powerful leading force behind the strong stance on the centrality of SRHR and women's equality. Fortunately, the group of "protesting" delegations and individuals at the Nairobi Summit was much smaller than expected and only nine countries ended up signing the U.S.-led statement.

THE IMPACT OF THE NOVEL CORONAVIRUS (COVID-19)

Only a few months after the Nairobi Conference, the world faced a horrific crisis: COVID-19. Since the World Health Organization declared the novel coronavirus a global pandemic in mid-March 2020, there has been an exponential increase in confirmed cases and deaths. By mid-August 2020, the number of reported COVID-19 cases globally had soared to over 20 million. The total number of deaths was close to 737,000. Approximately one-quarter of the reported cases and deaths occurred in the U.S although it represents only 4.25% of the world population. It is also deeply concerning that people of color in the U.S. have been disproportionately impacted by this pandemic.

We have never seen a disaster of this magnitude in our lifetime, affecting the lives and livelihoods of so many on this planet. This will have a profound impact on the achievement of the 2030 Sustainable Development goals. Health systems and providers are already stretched far beyond their capacity. Even in the wealthiest countries, including in the U.S., there have been shortages of test kits, personal protective equipment, ventilators, and other essential supplies and medicines to deal with COVID-19. In some places, there have not been enough health professionals or beds.

As this public health crisis continues to escalate in the U.S. and around the world, the biggest needs are increasingly in developing countries where the existing health infrastructure is already weak. This comes at a time when President Trump has cut off aid to the World Health Organization! During disasters, we always see a surge in the inequalities and suffering of women and adolescents along with poor, displaced, and other disadvantaged people throughout the developing world. In high density areas, such as urban slums and refugee camps, where social distancing is not possible, the risk of contracting the coronavirus is far greater. According to the U.N., there are approximately one billion people living in urban slums. They suffer from a lack of adequate shelter, health care, food, clean water, and basic sanitation. In sub-Saharan Africa, for example, one estimate indicates that only 15% of the population has access to clean water and soap.

The greatest fear is widespread hunger in developing countries as a result of COVID-19 and its sweeping health and economic consequences. Between 135 million and 265 million people could face severe hunger and starvation. There could be famine in over 30 countries. And we are seeing outbreaks of other diseases since vaccination programs have been disrupted. Related concerns are widespread riots and looting as meager incomes dry up. Emergency measures, in the form of cash transfers, are critical. The Group of 20 has pledged over $5 trillion to help those suffering from the pandemic. This will likely fall far short of meeting basic needs. One of the many constraining factors in responding to these emergencies is that the vital work of humanitarian organizations has been hampered due to insufficient supplies, staff layoffs, and the disruption of flights. In the 34 fragile and conflict-affected countries where it works, the International Rescue Committee has estimated that there could be up to one billion cases and 3.2 million deaths from COVID-19.

Along with the devastating global health and economic impact, the pandemic is severely crippling efforts to address the critical SRHR needs in every region. Individuals in developing countries are increasingly unable to exercise their basic human rights, such as obtaining contraceptives and safe abortion care plus other essential reproductive health services. There are many reasons why this is happening: home confinement, fear, the closure or repurposing of public and private health facilities, and shortages and reassignment of health care workers. The disruption of transportation, manufacturing and supply chains, and major stockouts are also contributing factors. In every developing country, we hear stories of women and girls suffering or dying from unsafe abortion because they could not access safe care, including medical abortion drugs and contraception.

India provides a dramatic example of how COVID-19 has severely disrupted women's access to safe abortion care. This is confirmed in a recent modelling exercise undertaken by Ipas Development Foundation (IDF) in India for the three-month period beginning with the country's lockdown on March 25, 2020. Of the 3.9 million abortions that would normally have taken place during this time, an estimated 1.85 million abortions (or 47%) were affected by the pandemic and confinement. Because of greatly reduced access to safe abortion through chemist outlets and public and private health facilities, women were faced with tough decisions. They were forced to choose from one of the following: delay seeking an abortion but ultimately obtain it from their preferred point of care, receive a surgical rather than a medical abortion (the preferred method of 80% of clients), undergo a second trimester abortion, continue their unintended pregnancy, or resort to an unsafe abortion. The IDF report *Compromised Abortion Access due to COVID-19* ends with a series of recommendations about how best to meet the needs of women now and in the future.

Other dimensions of the catastrophic impact of the novel coronavirus pandemic on SRHR include increased discrimination, domestic and partner violence, and sexual exploitation. At the end of April 2020, UNFPA released a shocking estimate of the likely increase in gender-based violence. It predicted an additional 31 million cases in 114 low-and middle-income countries if the lockdown continues for at least six months, and 15 million more for every three months of continuing quarantine. At the same time, there is decreased access to hotlines and vital peer and community support.

We know that a crisis of this magnitude will result in much higher levels of unsafe sex, sexually transmitted infections, unplanned and unintended pregnancies, unsafe abortion, and preventable deaths and disabilities. Guttmacher Institute researchers published in mid-April 2020 their analysis of the potential impact of COVID-19 on the sexual and reproductive health of individuals living in 132 low and middle-income countries around the world. Using a very conservative estimate of only a 10% proportional decrease during a 12-month period in the use of sexual and reproductive health care services in these countries, the impact is dramatic. There would be 49 million more women with an unmet need for modern contraception, 15 million additional unintended pregnancies, and 3.3 million more unsafe abortions leading to 1,000 more maternal deaths. In addition, a 10% reduction of essential pregnancy-related and newborn care would result in 1.7 million more women experiencing major obstetric complications and almost 2.6 million additional newborns with major complications. These combined complications would result in a death toll of another 196,000. The Guttmacher article notes, however, that partners on the ground feel that there could be a reduction of up to 80% of essential SRHR services, resulting in an extremely alarming scenario.

Since family planning, especially emergency contraception, and abortion care are time-sensitive services, it is imperative that online contraceptive information and counselling, and telemedicine for abortion with pills be made much more widely available. Medical abortion should be readily obtainable in local pharmacies and at other convenient points in communities. Where abortion services are not easily accessible, for a variety of reasons, women can safely end an unintended pregnancy at home, using a combination of mifepristone and misoprostol pills, with proper instruction and medical back up as needed. Women must also be able to obtain a contraceptive method of their choice to help prevent repeat abortions.

In its report on *Coronavirus disease (COVID-19) and Sexual and Reproductive Health*, the World Health Organization has categorized abortion as an essential service. Many countries around the world hold the same view on abortion, and efforts are underway to make it more widely accessible. Other countries, however, have done the opposite. In some cases, they are dramatically restricting the availability and use of abortion pills and are even prosecuting women for having an abortion. In the U.S., even though abortion is legal, some states have categorized abortion as "non-essential." Moreover, 18 states do not allow abortion care via telemedicine. Anti-abortion groups are actively involved in lobbying for these restrictive measures in the U.S. and in many other countries. Fortunately, there are organizations dedicated to helping women exercise their reproductive rights and are providing information and support online for safe pregnancy termination. But these organizations need substantially increased financial support.

At this time, we cannot predict the duration and full global impact of the COVID-19 pandemic. Nor do we know the timing and magnitude of a likely second wave of the virus or when an approved vaccine will be available. What is clear is that it will take a long time for individuals, nations, and economies to recover from this unprecedented crisis. The number of people living in poverty is soaring. And major gender and social inequalities are continuing to widen.

It is critical, especially in these tough times, that all partners increase support for key sexual and reproductive health services to the maximum extent possible and focus on the needs of the most vulnerable. In its late

April 2020 report, UNFPA indicated that its highest attention will be directed to "continuing sexual and reproductive health services and interventions, including protection of the health workforce; addressing gender-based violence; and ensuring the supply of modern contraceptives and reproductive health commodities."

The essential goals highlighted in the *Nairobi Statement on ICPD25* must receive the urgency they deserve from governments and non-governmental organizations, intergovernmental agencies, foundations, and the private sector. Equity in access, quality of care, and accountability are the key cross-cutting priorities to protect and achieve individuals' sexual and reproductive rights.

EXPANDING COVERAGE, USE, AND QUALITY OF SRH SERVICES

It is easy to feel overwhelmed by the enormity of the unmet needs in sexual and reproductive health, especially since they are rising dramatically as a result of COVID-19. However, we must put this in a broader perspective and recognize that we already have the knowledge and technologies to deal with most of these issues; and there are more innovations on the horizon.

To ensure that programs reach all who need SRH information and services, priority must be given to implementing integrated approaches to health care delivery. There must be new and innovative models of care, including those designed by and for youth. Women and girls need easy access to information about their bodies and their rights and how to prevent and manage safely unintended pregnancy.

Increasing the number of trained health care providers at all levels, especially mid-level providers and community health workers, is a tremendous challenge. Before COVID-19, the World Health Organization estimated that there would be a shortage of 18 million health workers by 2030! Now the shortfall is becoming even more acute. Currently, 70% of frontline health care providers and social workers are women.

Continued task-shifting and decentralization of services are essential along with expanded coverage and quality of care. To save and enhance people's lives, increased and sustained investments in health systems

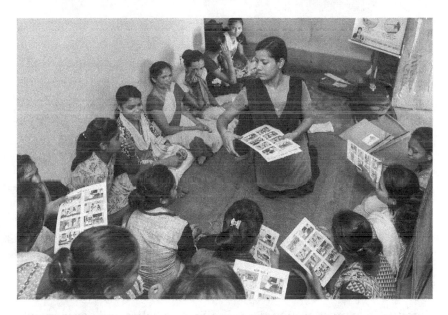

A youth leader conducting an outreach session on SRH issues with young women in Jharkhand, India. © IPAS DEVELOPMENT FOUNDATION (IDF)

improvements are desperately needed while ensuring, at the same time, uninterrupted availability of commodities and supplies as well as local transportation to health facilities. Reproductive health information hotlines and support networks require more funding as well.

Enhanced data collection, research, and analysis are also critical, along with prompt dissemination of findings, to inform policies and programs. Other priorities are scaling up cost-effective interventions, expanding the use of the latest technologies, and reaching the poor and marginalized populations, especially those at highest risk.

ACCELERATING ADVOCACY AND ENGAGEMENT

Achieving the ambitious goals that have been set and reiterated in the *Nairobi Statement on ICPD25* requires an urgent and increased mobilization of commitment and action at every level. Progress in each area of SRHR will have to occur at multiple times faster than at current levels, according to the 2018 Guttmacher-*Lancet* Commission report.

We need the advocacy and full engagement of an even broader representation of civil society—women's and youth groups, community organizations, health care officials and associations, along with human rights networks and coalitions, education and religious leaders, traditional leaders, and others. It is especially important to engage the talents and energy of young leaders at all levels, who represent the world's 1.8 billion young people. We count on their ideas and actions to help achieve the unfinished agenda.

Governments and the commercial sector must also provide greater leadership on these issues. We rely on governments to help assess supply and demand issues, prioritize interventions, and coordinate contributions to support SRH information and services. The commercial sector has a pivotal role to play as well.

At the same time, it is imperative that women and girls, together with other individuals—all working together—stand up and be heard. They must no longer be denied their choice, their health, and their human dignity. They must be empowered to hold societies and governments accountable for righting the wrongs of the past and enabling them to exercise their fundamental human rights. We must achieve a reality where women are co-equal members of all societies and where there is equity and equality in every aspect of life for people of all gender identities, ethnicities, and races.

REMOVING LEGAL, POLICY, SOCIOCULTURAL, AND OTHER BARRIERS

Governments and societies must take bold steps now to remove legal, policy, social, cultural, financial, and other barriers that stand in the way of individuals realizing their right to have control over their bodies and their lives. This requires effective multi-sectoral cooperation.

More information and education initiatives are needed, including extensive use of social media and the internet along with a greater focus on community-based activities. One example of an organization conducting innovative work in this area is IDF in India.

It is encouraging to see advances in addressing the stigma around issues like abortion, through the work of the INROADS initiative. The explosion of the #MeToo movement and sharing stories of sexual assault

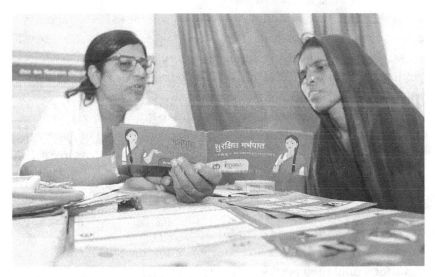

A health care provider counselling a client on comprehensive abortion care at a community health center in Madhya Pradesh, India. © IPAS DEVELOPMENT FOUNDATION (IDF)

and abuse are having a powerful impact in a growing number of countries.

Other efforts to address sociocultural barriers are proving to be effective as well. However, so much more must be done throughout the developing world to change social and gender norms, laws, policies, and practices. This is especially critical in the area of abortion, where efforts to reform restrictive laws and policies must be accelerated to respond to women's needs for safe, legal, and comprehensive abortion care, including contraception.

Overcoming the intense political and religious opposition to abortion in countries around the world is an ongoing battle. We must use the lessons from the COVID-19 pandemic to advocate strongly for changes, including greater availability of telemedicine for medical abortion as well as self-managed care.

INCREASING POLITICAL WILL AND RESOURCES

The greatest challenge is how to dramatically increase political will and resources for sexual and reproductive health at a time when national governments and foreign donors have not kept up with previous pledges and growing demand in the face of many competing priorities. The needs are especially acute at this time given the immense suffering and havoc caused by the COVID-19 pandemic. As early as March 2020, UNFPA estimated that it needed $187.5 million just to fund its response to the current public health emergency in the most vulnerable settings. This number will continue to rise.

Even in the present crisis, it is important to note that the costs of SRH information and services are more affordable compared to many other areas of needed investment. We also know that investments in SRH are essential to the achievement of health, human rights, and sustainable development goals and that they yield enormous dividends over many generations.

The 2018 Guttmacher-*Lancet* Commission provided global estimates to meet the unmet need for core components of the SRH agenda. At that time, for a minimum package of contraception, abortion, and maternal and newborn health information and services, the total cost was estimated at $54 billion a year for low and middle-income countries, or $9 per capita a year. These three interventions are particularly cost-effective in reducing health care costs and freeing up scarce resources.

In preparation for the Nairobi Summit, UNFPA and several partner organizations estimated that by 2030, in 120 priority countries, $115.5 billion would be required to end preventable maternal deaths and $68.5 billion to eliminate unmet needs for family planning. For another set of priority countries, $79.4 billion is required to end gender-based violence and other harmful practices. Achieving these three goals totals $263.4 billion. The current investment is approximately $42 billion, leaving a gap of almost $222 billion. As a result of the current global health crisis, these estimates will have to be revised.

By the end of the Nairobi Summit in November 2019, 1,500 commitments were made, totaling billions of dollars in pledges. In the coming years, as countries try to mobilize from all sources the necessary funding for SRH information and services, the corporate sector and social entrepreneurs must play a much more significant role. The *Nairobi Statement on ICPD25: Accelerating the Promise* called for increased domestic and international financing along with "exploring new, participatory and innovative financing instruments and structures." The International Monetary Fund and the World Bank are key actors, along with greatly expanded health insurance, as governments strive to achieve the goal of universal health coverage. Unfortunately, COVID-19 is substantially hindering these efforts. In April 2020, the World Bank committed $160 billion to respond to the pandemic. But we do not know when and how many resources will be directed to meeting SRH needs.

The work of international and local NGO partners, dependent on donor support, has become much more challenging, especially since the outbreak of the novel coronavirus. In the last few years, NGOs have been dealing with an increasingly competitive environment, more complex and demanding donor requirements, and changing funding priorities. With this global pandemic, endowments are plummeting and uncertainties about future donor funding are rising. At a minimum, many NGOs have had to make steep cuts in staff and programs; an unknown number may have to close their operations.

And yet, the full engagement and collaboration of *all* partners and multiple sectors, along with global and regional alliances, are crucial to meet the daunting task of massive resource mobilization for sexual and reproductive health and rights and to ensure the effective utilization of funds.

With the devastation caused by the global coronavirus pandemic and other disasters that are likely to follow, it is hard to imagine that the ambitious SRHR and other critical 2030 Sustainable Development Goals can be met a decade from now. However, we must ensure that there is greatly accelerated progress in the coming years and that these goals will *ultimately* be achieved!

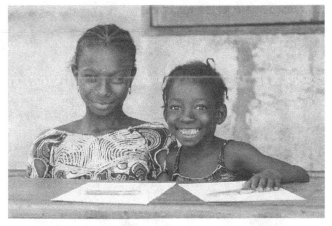

Ensuring fundamental rights for future generations. SHUTTERSTOCK

PART FIVE

MAXIMIZING LIFE'S OPPORTUNITIES

MEMORABLE AND REWARDING EXPERIENCES

16

FOLLOWING MY PASSIONS

It is not the years in your life but the life in your years that counts.

— ADLAI STEVENSON

At my retirement party in June 2015, former Ipas Board Chair Amy Tsui gave me a wooden sign that reads: She Designed a Life She Loved. It is hanging on the wall of my study at home, and I often smile at how accurate a reflection this is of my life and how grateful I am for all that I have learned and experienced, with the love and support of my family and friends.

Adjusting to retirement, or semi-retirement, was initially challenging after an enormously stimulating career of 45 years. As a real extrovert, I was very energized by working all day with wonderful people on a common mission, even when it meant that there was not much time for non-work-related activities.

In the beginning, I had to adopt a different daily rhythm as well as spend time dealing with some health issues that I had neglected for many years during my career. While this was frustrating, I was determined not to have them dominate my days. I believe that having a positive attitude is critical to maintaining a happy and fulfilling life. There are always new experiences and adventures ahead. I am focused on making the most of life's opportunities even in the grim context of COVID-19, where physical distancing is especially difficult for someone who thrives on social interaction.

I am still spending time on my lifelong passion of helping women in developing countries realize their reproductive health, rights, and full potential in life. Now I am doing this at a reduced level and more relaxed pace. I have been making contributions through Board service, mentoring aspiring young professionals, supporting former colleagues as they advance in their careers, keeping up with the latest developments in my field, speaking at various events, and writing. These activities will always be important to me.

While continuing to follow advances in my former institutions and those of many partner organizations, I recently served for four years as a Board member of Pathfinder International. Founded in 1957, Pathfinder is "driven by the conviction that all people, regardless of where they live, have the right to decide whether and when to have children, to exist free from fear and stigma, and to lead the lives they choose." The organization enhances the reproductive health and rights of women and adolescents by expanding access to high-quality contraception and safe abortion care as well as to maternal, neonatal, and other services. They reach some of the most vulnerable populations through their support of public health systems and local communities. Pathfinder is doing pioneering work to inform and empower young people to have control over their reproductive lives and to address the nexus of population, health, and climate resilience, among other areas of focus.

Most of all, I appreciate the opportunity to be a "thought partner" and mentor to others in the SRHR field who are in different countries around the world. With email, Skype, What's App, and Zoom, there are virtually no barriers of time or distance. The conversations are always stimulating and a source of inspiration for me.

Enjoying Time with Family and Friends

I love having more time with Terry, family, and friends. While I sometimes regret that we do not have our own children and grandchildren, we are fortunate to have other family members of all ages. It is also nice to keep up with the children and grandchildren of friends.

I have been able to spend more quality moments, in person and virtually, with my siblings, Stephanie and Henry, and their spouses. Moreover, it is gratifying to watch my niece, Liz, and nephew, Chris, and their spouses lead busy and rewarding lives. My other nephew, Stuart, is only

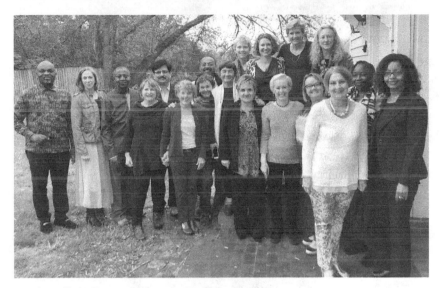

Reunion of Ipas Alums and Country Directors, 2018.

a teenager and has many productive years ahead. I am so proud of all of them. We have the added pleasure of following the next generation, my great-niece and four great-nephews, who are smart, gifted, and pursuing their own interests. The only downside is that we live in different parts of the country.

Another wonderful aspect of retirement is the chance to reconnect with friends around the world, many of whom are former USAID and Ipas colleagues. In 2018, we had a marvelous reunion in Chapel Hill of seven Ipas Country Directors and members of the Ipas alums group who live nearby. We all had fun reminiscing and catching up.

While many of my close friends are no longer working, we have schedules that fill up with a variety of activities. For those in the Chapel Hill area, our visits have been mostly replaced by phone calls as we observe physical distancing and social solidarity during the COVID-19 pandemic. I miss regular outings and exchanging hugs with special people.

Since I retired, I have also enjoyed seeing my old college friend, Jodie, who lives five minutes away. It is hard to believe that we have known each other for over 50 years, especially when we can't possibly look a half-century older! When we are not travelling, Jodie and I try to see each other regularly for a couple of hours and talk about what is happening in our lives, including the latest books we have read. The time passes all too quickly. We could easily spend the whole day together and never run out of topics to discuss. For the period of confinement, we have been limited to catching up virtually.

There are other college friends, Bonnie and Judith, as well as my high school friend, Jill, with whom I enjoy staying in touch although we live too far apart to see each often. I had hoped to visit each of them in 2020 along with my dear friends in New York, Barbara, and Mary, but all travel plans are on hold until next year at the earliest. I look forward to seeing many friends and former colleagues in the Washington, D.C. area as well in 2021.

FEEDING MY MIND AND BODY

Another critical part of my life is reading, exercising, and eating well—all vital to my mental and physical well-being. Retirement has provided new opportunities to stretch my mind and body and focus on improving my microbiome as well as engage more in hobbies, see movies, listen to music, and continue my path of personal growth and "giving back."

The joy of reading: My Kindle is my constant companion, enhancing my knowledge, critical thinking, and perspectives. Every night, I read for 45 minutes to an hour before going to sleep. I always look forward to delving into another interesting book. The ones I select are generally from *The New York Times* Best Sellers List, and those recommended by friends as well as books in French that are not on my Kindle. I tend to gravitate more towards nonfiction, with many books covering the period of World War II in France and the resistance movement. This long-time interest stems from all the stories I heard from my French cousins who lived during this period. Now these books seem more relevant as we fight our own war against COVID-19.

Among the latest books I have read on this topic are Erik Larson's *The Splendid and the Vile: A Saga of Churchill, Family,* and *Defiance During the Blitz* and Lynne Olson's *Madame Fourcade's Secret War: The Daring Young Woman Who Led France's Largest Spy Network Against Hitler. A Woman of No Importance: The Untold Story of the American Spy Who Helped Win World*

War II by Sonia Purnell was fascinating as well. There is also *Unbroken: A World War II Story of Survival, Resilience, and Redemption* by Laura Hillenbrand, and *A Train in Winter: An Extraordinary Story of Women, Friendship, and Resistance in Occupied France* by Caroline Moorehead. Another one I enjoyed was Agnès Poirier's account of the life of famous philosophers, writers, artists, and musicians in Paris during and after the Second World War, entitled *Left Bank: Art, Passion, and the Rebirth of Paris, 1940–1950*.

Other books that have captured my interest recount the lives of great leaders such as Presidents Lincoln, Roosevelt, Obama, and Mandela. I was touched by the deep friendship and shared values of His Holiness the 14th Dalai Lama and Archbishop Desmond Tutu in *The Book of Joy: Lasting Happiness in a Changing World*, co-written with Douglas Abrams. One of my all-time favorite books is Michelle Obama's *Becoming*. I recently finished reading Eddie Glaude Jr.'s *Begin Again: James Baldwin's America and Its Urgent Lessons for Our Own*. I have more books to read on my Kindle on systemic racism and social injustice in the U.S.

I have also learned a lot from Jon Meacham's books, including *Songs of America* and *The Soul of America*, as well as Madeleine Albright's *Fascism: A Warning* and *Hell and Other Destinations: A 21st-Century Memoir*. I was captivated by Trevor Noah's *Born a Crime: Stories from a South African Childhood*, William Kamkwamba's *The Boy Who Harnessed the Wind*, Ruth Bader Ginsburg's *My Own Words*, Samantha Power's *The Education of an Idealist: A Memoir*, and Rachel Maddow's *Blowout*. Other interesting and carefully researched books include Anthony Shadid's *House of Stone: A Memoir of Home, Family, and a Lost Middle East* as well as *The Seine: The River that Made Paris* by Elaine Sciolino.

In terms of fiction, I enjoy reading periodically Nicolas Sparks's books, which are based in North Carolina, and occasionally mysteries written by Mary Higgins Clark and John Le Carré. One of the best books I have ever read is Amor Towles's *A Gentleman in Moscow: A Novel*, where I dwelled on every line and had to be disciplined not to read it all at once.

I have expanded my knowledge by reading books on health, such as Dr. William W. Li's *Eat to Beat Disease: The New Science of How Your Body Can Heal Itself*, and Dr. Amy Myers's *The Autoimmune Solution: Prevent and Reverse the Full Spectrum of Inflammatory Symptoms and Diseases*.

Another fascinating book, on a totally different subject, is *The Genius of Birds* by Jennifer Ackerman. Also remarkable is Richard Powers's *The Overstory: A Novel.* As a lifelong dog lover, I obtained new information and pleasure from the book *Inside of a Dog: What Dogs See, Smell, and Know* by Alexandra Horowitz. Her latest book is on my Kindle.

Of course, I always look forward to reading books related to women's health, rights, and empowerment, such as Cecile Richards's *Make Trouble: Standing up, Speaking Out, and Finding the Courage to Lead—My Life Story* as well as Melinda Gates's *The Moment of Lift: How Empowering Women Changes the World,* and Merle Hoffman's *Intimate Wars.* I also appreciated *Champion of Choice: The Life and Legacy of Women's Advocate Nafis Sadik* by Cathleen Miller.

The rewards of exercising: For basic exercise, Terry and I enjoy our daily walks. In Chapel Hill, we like talking to neighborhood friends, while maintaining a proper distance, and engaging with all the friendly dogs we pass as well as watching and listening to the many species of birds in the area. This is a time for us to discuss a wide range of topics. On the other side of the Atlantic, we do a lot more walking while admiring spectacular vistas.

I also have a series of stretching and strengthening exercises that I do at home. Going through these daily, however, requires a lot of discipline and is often displaced by other activities. In the last several years, I have appreciated the value of yoga and doing relaxation exercises that I should have done during all the years when I was working, but never seemed to find the time for these beneficial activities.

Healthy eating: After four decades of suffering from too many bad bacteria, parasites, and antibiotics, I finally turned to the task of addressing my gastrointestinal problems. In addition to following herbal treatment regimens to improve the functioning of my gut, I radically changed my diet to a diverse, healthy one of fish, chicken and some beef, along with a wide range of vegetables and fruit while eliminating gluten, dairy, sugar, and soy.

I wondered whether I would be able to make these big adjustments, including cutting out all the desserts I love. To my surprise, it has been easier than I expected. Terry is a creative chef and has even managed to satisfy my sweet tooth with cookies made with non-gluten flours, coconut, and cacao as well as non-dairy ice cream filled with cacao chips. I can even eat 100% dark chocolate, so life is good! The benefit of these changes is that my microbiome is improving substantially.

17

LIVING IN FRANCE

The most exciting part of this latest chapter in my life is spending more time in France where Terry and I have a small *pied-à-terre*. When we decided to put down roots outside the U.S. 35 years ago, I was able to realize a dream that started in my adolescence. As Terry and I began our search, we established three criteria to determine the location: a cosmopolitan city in France with many cultural attractions, an area with an abundance of sun throughout the year, and a place near Italy. The city that met these criteria was Nice (population of 350,000, with a larger metropolitan area of one million people). Nice is in the southeast corner of France, eight miles from Monaco and 19 miles from the Italian border.

This area is one of the oldest in Europe where stone tools have been discovered dating from one million years ago. Nice was named after the Greek word Nikaia (the Goddess of Victory) in the 4th century B.C. when the Greeks dominated the area, followed by the Roman, Saracen, and Ottoman empires. Beginning in the Middle Ages, for close to 500 years, Nice was under the control of the Kingdom of Savoy and then was part of the Kingdom of Piedmonte-Sardinia until it reverted back to France in 1860. The city became famous following an influx of English aristocrats, including Queen Victoria in the late 19th century, and wealthy Russians and northern Europeans who wanted to escape the cold weather. Because of its mild climate, plenty of sun, and special light, many famous artists flocked to Nice, including Henri Matisse and Marc Chagall. Pierre-Auguste Renoir and Pablo Picasso lived for periods of time in nearby towns.

Beginning in the mid-1980s, we spent our annual vacations in a tiny two-room garden apartment (323 sq. feet) on the eastern edge of Nice,

650 feet above the port, with a panoramic view of the mountains and sea. The only problem was during the hottest days of the summer. With no cross ventilation and a small, noisy air conditioning unit, we found it challenging to sleep. The plus side of the apartment was that we never had to worry about anything when we left for prolonged periods. We developed a close friendship with our French neighbors in the adjacent apartment who deepened our appreciation of the local culture and introduced us to many attractions in the area. Our Italian neighbors on the other side became good friends as well.

Our Renovation Experience

Two decades ago, we purchased in the same neighborhood in Nice a small dilapidated house built in 1932, which had received little in the way of upgrading for many decades. As a result, the price of the house was much reduced and affordable compared to others in the area.

Before we were able to live there, we had to undertake a complete renovation. This involved installing a septic tank; replacing all the pipes and electrical wires; tearing down walls; and adding insulation, new floors, ceilings, windows, shutters, and doors. We also had to put in a new heating and air conditioning system; build a new kitchen, bathrooms and closets; turn the old garage into a tiny guest suite; add new stucco and paint; and create a small garden out of a mass of weeds. The renovation took four times as long to complete as a similar job in the U.S. Of course, there wasn't much incentive for the team to work when we were on the other side of the Atlantic. This multi-year experience was a big adventure, full of frustrations and setbacks but ultimately well worth it and a great joy.

Having read Peter Mayle's books (including *A Year in Provence* and *Toujours Provence*) about renovating his house in Provence, Terry and I pondered whether we should write one about our own challenges in Nice. Even after we moved from our apartment into our newly renovated house, we continued to deal with a lot of issues. Had we decided to write a book, the words "septic tank" or "sewer" might have been in the title because the most pressing concern we faced had to do with the newly installed *fausse septique*, which was transmitting too many odors in parts of the house. It took over a year of detective work and repair to fix the problem. Soon

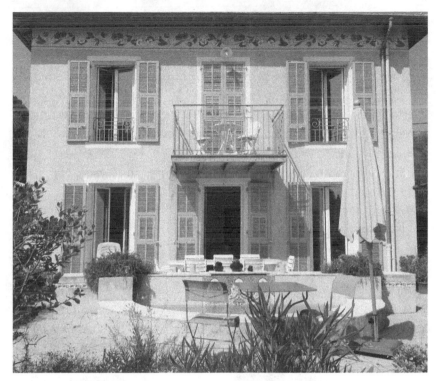

Our house after renovation, 2015

afterwards, municipal authorities finally got around to connecting our neighborhood to the Nice sewer system. All the time and money we spent on this problem was wasted except for the adventures we experienced.

Other house-related issues in recent years have included buying all new aluminum shutters since the wooden ones were attacked by carpenter bees. We also had to upgrade the sprinkler system, change all the interior lights to LED fixtures and bulbs, install a new alarm system, and replace the hot water system and the air conditioning units. Among the remaining jobs is repairing part of the exterior walls of the house as well as repainting the façade and interior. The biggest task that lies ahead is replacing the nearly 90-year-old tile roof, an expensive, month-long undertaking, if all goes smoothly.

Much of the work we have done to date is what many homeowners experience. However, doing major house repairs in the south of France adds more time and unique challenges. In the process, we have worked with a fascinating group of tradespeople—from different skills, backgrounds, and countries of origin—leaving us with some unforgettable memories. One tip we picked up was that offering the workers *un petit café* provided an impetus for them to work even harder. In fact, the more frequently we made this offer, the happier they were. We also learned to stay out of their way as much as possible except to welcome each worker with a warm "Bonjour" at the beginning of the day and provide an appreciative "Merci infiniment" once the job was completed.

The one sad development is that the architect who worked with us on our house for several years died recently of COVID-19.

Making the Most of Every Day

Before retiring in 2015, we spent two to four weeks a year in Nice. Since then, we have lived up to half of each year overseas, although this has changed in 2020 as a result of the novel coronavirus. Terry adores working in the garden that surrounds our small house. He takes care of the flowers, abundant supply of herbs, our olivier, and several fruit trees. He also keeps the rapidly growing bushes and vines trimmed and the tenacious weeds under control as well as oversees repairs needed inside and outside the house. Moreover, Terry does the food shopping and is a master chef. How could I be so lucky!

My responsibility has been more on the decorating and event planning side, including having a colorful house bathed in yellows and blues with interesting pictures on the walls and Italian, Provençal, and Tunisian ceramics inside and out. I also spend many hours during each visit researching all the cultural attractions in the Alpes-Maritimes department (in the southeast corner of France) and organizing our social schedule, which is especially busy in the summer months. Even at the beginning of 2020, we managed to attend many concerts and movies during a six-week period before there was a moratorium on public events and we had to return to the U.S. given the expanding public health crisis. Now it is not certain when we will be able to go back to France.

While in Nice, we love living outdoors as much as possible, especially when the bougainvillea, jasmine, lavender, morning glories, and other plants are in bloom. We enjoy dining at our beautiful table in the garden,

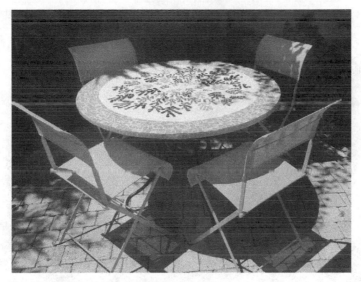

Our Matisse-inspired table, 2018

which was a surprise gift from my Executive Team at Ipas when I retired. Terry found an artist in Vieux Nice who was able to produce a mosaic tabletop inspired by one of my favorite Matisse paintings (*La Gerbe*) where the predominant colors are blue, yellow, and green.

We share our garden with a pair of turtle doves and other species of birds, including a family of blackbirds who nest in the hedges. The male blackbird has a large repertoire of songs that he performs throughout the day and into the evening during the mating season. The seagulls flying overhead are a welcome sight along with the swallows at dusk. In the summertime we listen to the cicadas during the day and evening and the frogs at night. We also have beautiful butterflies and bees along with mosquitos during the summer who seem only interested in me. Using plenty of insect repellant helps.

Every day we like to walk on one of the trails near our house, especially one that winds around the Cap de Nice with stunning vistas to the west of the Bay of Angels, the port, and city of Nice along with the vast stretch of sea to the south. Looking to the east on our walk, there is a spectacular panorama of the Bay of Villefranche, Saint-Jean-Cap-Ferrat, and the mountains and water stretching to Monaco. On a really clear day, we occasionally see the island of Corsica.

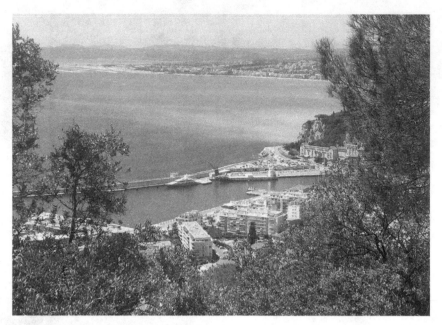

View of Nice and the Bay of Angels, 2018

The municipal park of Mont Boron covers an area of over 165 acres with almost seven miles of walking trails. It is full of Aleppo pines, carob, and wild olive trees, and a rich and varied vegetation of cactus and other plants. At the north end of the park on Mont Boron, just beyond Elton John's sumptuous villa, is a 16th-century fort with more magnificent views, including one overlooking the seaside town of Villefranche-sur-Mer far below.

We are fortunate to be the only Americans in our quartier. Over the years, we have made wonderful friends, mostly French and Italian. Our next-door neighbors, Alex and Annie, were always extremely warm, welcoming, and generous from the time we bought and renovated the house twenty years ago. We would talk over the fence almost every day and loved seeing the "quatre pattes" (the dogs) as well. We have spent many delightful Sunday afternoons at their house with the family gathered around the table for a delicious lunch and lively conversation lasting at least four hours. It was heartbreaking to learn of the sudden death of Annie in April of this year, soon after we returned to the U.S. from our last visit. We will miss her greatly and wish we could be in Nice to support the

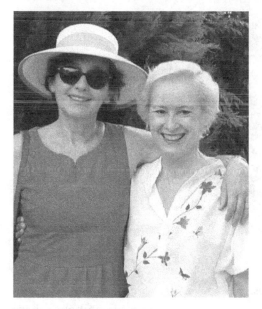

With my friend Odile, 2018

family during this painful period. We are staying in touch through regular phone calls.

Other close French friends are retired teachers who live just three blocks away—Odile and Alain—with whom we enjoy going to concerts, movies, and on other interesting outings. Odile and I have become soulmates, with similar personalities and interests. Although we have lived in the same neighborhood for decades, we only met five years ago and have been making up for lost time. We have spent many delightful moments together and look forward to more ahead, post the COVID-19 pandemic.

NOURISHING MY SOUL

Music is the social act of communication among people, a gesture of friendship, the strongest there is.

— MALCOLM ARNOLD

Being in Nice in the summer and attending outdoor concerts has always been exhilarating. Listening to music became a great passion of mine in my later years, following almost 10 years of piano lessons when I was in my youth. We have regularly attended the free Sunday afternoon performance of the Orchestre d'Harmonie (a 50-member orchestra of mostly woodwind, brass, and percussion instruments), which plays during the summer in a large olive grove next to the Matisse Museum and the ruins of a Roman amphitheater. We arrive an hour early, with reading materials in hand, in order to grab front row seats. By doing so, we get the most out of each concert and can talk to our musician friends afterwards.

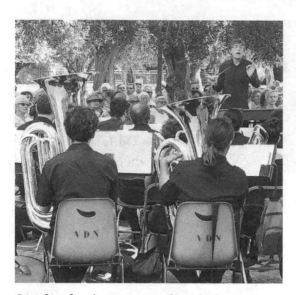

One of our favorite summer pastimes, 2019

Terry particularly enjoys listening to the tuba since he played this instrument during high school. The rest of the year the orchestra performs in the church at the head of the Port of Nice, down the hill from where we live. We also attend performances of the Philharmonic Orchestras of Nice, Monte-Carlo, and Cannes-PACA—all within an hour's drive from our house. In the summer, there are musical evenings in a broad array of settings, including in the stained glass auditorium of the Chagall Museum, the magnificent courtyard of the Palace in Monaco, and the open-air theater in Villefranche-sur-Mer, where we overlook the water on one side and the ramparts of the 16th-century citadel on the other. We have especially enjoyed going to the annual International Mandolin Festival in the mountain village of Castellar near the Italian border. Thank goodness Terry is an experienced mountain driver because there are endless hairpin turns along the narrow steep road to Castellar.

During the summer there are free concerts in practically every town along the Mediterranean in this part of France and in almost every medieval village perched in the mountains. The music ranges from classical to jazz, rock, country, soul, and polyphonic songs from Corsica. All this is food for my soul! I am lucky that Terry enjoys these events as well. It's fun to share these concerts with family and friends when they visit.

Due to COVID-19, most concerts in the region have been postponed or cancelled for the summer of 2020. We hope this will change in 2021, although the experience will probably never be the same with social distancing regulations. For now, we are enjoying concerts online, which provide a source of comfort during a stressful time.

Fascinating Places to Visit

Spending part of the year in Nice has been an experience of continuous discovery and adventure. We enjoy the beauty of the Mediterranean Sea only a short car or bus ride away as well as the fascinating villages in the mountains in our area. Other main attractions are the lively open-air markets and local food specialties, and the many interesting sites and museums. All this is in addition to the huge variety of cultural events throughout the year.

Nice: We have never run out of things to do in Nice and love spending time downtown, strolling through le Vieux-Nice with its medieval streets, narrow multistoried houses with pastel façades, many churches and restaurants, and art galleries. There is also a wide variety of small clothing and food shops, including one featuring spices, salt, and pepper from around the world. A trip to Old Nice always includes a stop at the colorful food and flower market in the famous Cours Saleya just a block from the sea. At one end of the long courtyard is the magnificent Opéra de Nice where we have attended many concerts. Up a steep hill from Old Nice is the "Château" first occupied by the Greeks and later the site of a huge fortress during the Middle Ages, which was subsequently destroyed.

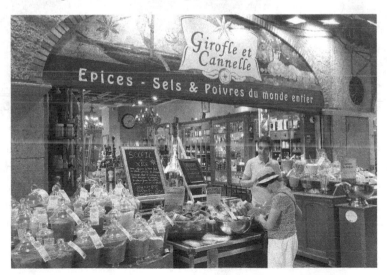

Shopping in Old Nice with my friends Mary and Barbara, 2018

Nice is France's largest tourist resort on the water. The famous Promenade des Anglais along the Baie des Anges (Bay of Angels) is lined with the city's trademark *chaises bleues* and palm trees. At the east end of the four-mile seaside walkway is one of my favorite landmarks that captures how I feel about Nice.

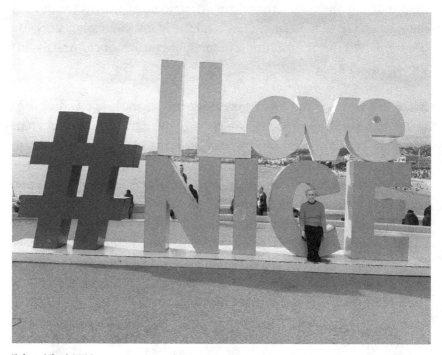

J'aime Nice! 2020

The architecture of Nice is interesting and varied with many grand Belle Époque buildings. More recent additions to the city include a beautiful park that runs from the Museum of Modern Art through the heart of Nice to the waterfront. There are fountains, gardens, and playgrounds for kids and families. One of Nice's landmarks is the Place Masséna, a spacious square designed in the mid-19th century. It is surrounded on the north end by majestic red ochre buildings with archways and modern statues perched on high pillars. A huge fountain sits on the south side of the square featuring a giant marble statue of Apollo surrounded by five smaller bronze statues.

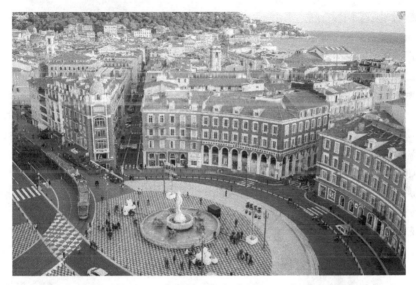

Place Masséna with Old Nice and the sea in the background. ISTOCK.COM / IALF

Another marvelous feature of Nice is the relatively new tramway system, which traverses large areas of the city and now extends from the Port at the bottom of our hill to the airport, about five miles away. Nice is also home to many interesting museums, including those dedicated to the life and works of Marc Chagall and Henri Matisse.

West of Nice: Provence is only two hours away, with all its attractions and rich history dating back to prehistoric times. In addition to the fascinating city of Marseille (population of 1.6 million), there are the Roman cities of Aix, Avignon, and Arles as well as some charming smaller towns and villages such as Gordes, Roussillon, Saint-Rémy-de-Provence, and L'Isle-sur-la-Sorgue. There are endless fields of lavender and sunflowers to admire, along with the rugged landscape, stone houses, excellent wines and perfumes, and a wide array of cultural events, especially during the summer.

Saint-Tropez on the French Riviera attracts the "rich and famous" but is not a place where we want to spend any time. An hour from Nice is Cannes, home to the "stars," with its renowned annual international film festival that started in 1946. Cannes is also known for its Belle Époque architecture, fancy hotels, elegant stores, and beautiful beaches.

Closer to Nice is Antibes, a much smaller and more interesting place on the water. Its newest port is reportedly the largest yachting haven in Europe. The old town is full of quaint stores, restaurants, and a large covered market as well as the lovely Picasso Museum in the Château Grimaldi facing the sea. At different times, the area in and around Antibes featured celebrities such as Guy de Maupassant, Victor Hugo, Rudolf Valentino, Ernest Hemingway, and F. Scott Fitzgerald as well as former King Edward VIII and Wallis, Duchess of Windsor. Another popular area is Saint-Paul-de-Vence. This perched medieval village has been visited, over many decades, by a wide array of artists, actors, writers, and tourists.

East of Nice: We like to spend most of our time in areas east of Nice, wandering through the villages in the mountains between Nice and the Italian border as well as the lovely towns along the coast.

Closest to our house is the picturesque seaside town of Villefranche-sur-Mer which straddles the western side of one of the deepest bays in the Mediterranean. The Russian Navy had a base here in the late 19th century as did the U.S. Sixth Fleet in the 20th century (1950–1966). Now the bay serves as a port of call for large cruise ships. There is a nice selection of restaurants along the waterfront and a lovely beach. The most dramatic landmark is the 16th-century citadel, featured in at least one James Bond movie. It currently houses the town hall, several interesting museums,

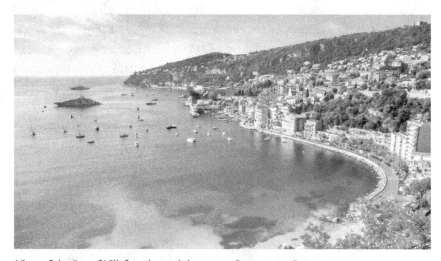

View of the Bay of Villefranche and the town. ISTOCK.COM / BARETA

and a spectacular open-air theater next to the water where we see movies and concerts during the summer. We also love walking through the town's steep narrow streets and along the old harbor of La Darse, built in the 17th century where the oceanographic observatory is also located.

On the other side of the Bay of Villefranche is Saint-Jean-Cap-Ferrat, with some of the most expensive real estate in the world. It has served as home to many celebrities in the past, including Charlie Chaplin, David Niven, W. Somerset Maugham, and Édith Piaf. Winston Churchill, Rudyard Kipling, Ian Fleming, T.S. Eliot, and Virginia Woolf also spent time in this stunning area. Today, many wealthy people reside in Saint-Jean-Cap-Ferrat at least part of the year. The lovely harbor of St. Jean is worth a visit. If you follow the coastal path that winds around the peninsula, you can admire the sumptuous estates and the breathtaking vistas of the Mediterranean, including the Bay of Villefranche. We like to attend summer evening concerts at the Villa Ephrussi de Rothschild, where we enjoy the music while visiting the spectacular gardens and fountains and appreciating the backdrop of the mountains and sea.

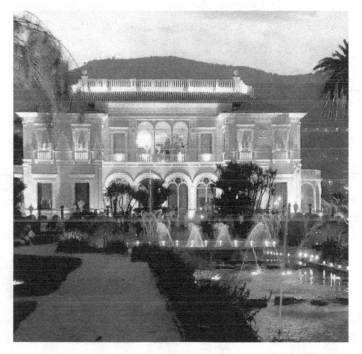

Attending an evening concert at the Villa Ephrussi de Rothschild, 2019

Another charming seaside town, only a ten-minute drive from our house, is Beaulieu-sur-Mer, with its lush vegetation and manicured gardens, beautiful hotels and beaches, and large yacht harbor lined with restaurants. One of the famous landmarks is the Villa Kérylos, built in the style of an ancient Greek villa a little over a hundred years ago and now a museum. It was the site of the 2019 dinner hosted by President Macron of France for President Xi of China. We have enjoyed some delightful evenings listening to concerts in the central courtyard of the villa on the waterfront. Like other towns in this area, Beaulieu-sur-Mer attracted many celebrities, including Gustave Eiffel, the famous architectural engineer. Another important person who lived in Beaulieu in a mansion with views of the sea and his yacht was James Gordon Bennett, Jr., the flamboyant publisher who launched the *International Herald Tribune* in Paris.

When President Obama visited Èze-Village with his family in the summer of 2019, he commented, according to the newspaper *Nice Matin*, "It is the most spectacular village I have ever seen." Èze-Village is perched on a rocky cliff 1,400 feet above the seaside town of Èze-sur-Mer where the singer Bono resides. You can climb all the way from the water's edge along Le Chemin de Nietzsche (named after the philosopher who loved

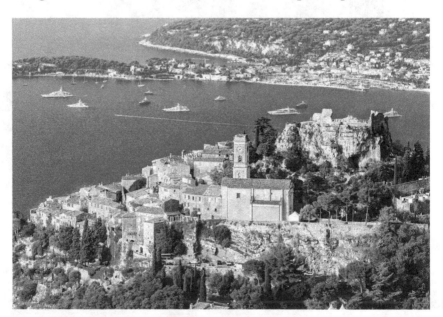

The spectacular village of Èze. iStock.com / Lucentius

this area) to Èze-Village. After completing the ascent for the first time, Nietzsche commented, "I laughed a lot and I found a marvelous vigor and patience." It was the inspiration for one of his books. There is an easier route to the top of Èze from the parking lot below, although it is still a steep walk up to the top. The climb is well worth it, because there is a beautiful cactus garden at the summit where you can enjoy sensational views of the surrounding mountains, coastal towns, and the Mediterranean Sea.

La Turbie is another pleasant town that is perched on top of the Grande Corniche (the highest mountain road) overlooking Monaco far below. The most interesting attraction is the Trophée des Alpes built by the Romans in the 6th century B.C. to mark the frontier between Italy and Gaul. The poet Dante was one of many who have found this giant monument inspiring.

Monaco was initially a Greek and then a Roman colony. It has been a principality since the beginning of the 14th century and is the smallest sovereign state in the world after the Vatican. It covers an area of .8 square miles, only 60% of New York City's Central Park. It has the world's highest per capita income with slightly over 38,000 inhabitants representing 140 nationalities. Most of the residents live in skyscraper buildings. Major landmarks include the Prince's Palace, the Oceanographic Museum, the Casino, and the Exotic Garden. Terry and I would never want to live there but will drive the 30 minutes from our house to attend performances of the renowned Monte-Carlo Philharmonic Orchestra.

Another fun place to visit is Menton on the border with Italy. It is known as the *perle de la France* and the lemon festival capital of the world. Menton is a beautiful town on the water with many Belle Époque buildings and a charming old section. It has a mild climate where you can swim in the sea and ski in the mountains the same day. It is home to some lovely gardens open to the public and to the museum dedicated to Jean Cocteau, the famous poet, artist, and filmmaker. Menton also features the Mirazur restaurant, which reached in 2019 the top spot on the World's Best Restaurants list.

18

ADVENTURES IN
OTHER COUNTRIES

MEDITERRANEAN MARVELS

Italy: Our second great love is Italy, which we visit whenever possible. The first large town across the French border is Ventimiglia, which takes less than an hour to reach from our house. There, we can shop in the outdoor markets, eat a leisurely lunch, and stroll along the waterfront. I also enjoy the chance to speak Italian.

There are so many spectacular places to explore in Italy. Together, we have toured large sections of both coasts and have visited most of the country's 20 regions. Of course, a highlight for us is Tuscany. We have been back several times to Firenze (my home in 1968) and other wonderful attractions in the area. Tuscany is deservedly a popular tourist destination with its rich history, art, culture, museums, churches, music, wines, cuisine, and textiles. Moreover, the region has beautiful landscapes and nature reserves. In addition to all the marvels of Firenze, the birthplace of the Renaissance, there are many other enticing towns throughout Tuscany. My favorites include Siena, San Gimignano, Pisa, Arezzo, Montepulciano, Lucca, and Castiglione della Pescaia on the Mediterranean.

We have some close friends in Spoleto and Torino, which are fascinating places to visit along with all the major attractions in Rome, Venice, Milano and other magnificent cities. We love the Lake District in the northwestern part of the country and look forward to spending more time in Sicily as well.

Fascinating islands: Over the years, we have had a chance to visit some of the amazing islands in the Mediterranean Sea, which covers a vast area of almost one million square miles, stretching from the Atlantic Ocean to the Middle East and from Southern Europe and Western Turkey to North Africa .

One of our favorite spots is the island of Corsica, 124 miles southeast of Nice. Colonized by the Greeks and Romans and then occupied for centuries by other external powers, Corsica experienced a brief period of independence beginning in 1755. During that time, it took the bold move of giving women the right to vote. Corsica was sold to France in 1768. Following the French Revolution and a period of union with Great Britain, the island returned to French rule in 1796. Nevertheless, it proudly maintains its language, traditions, and spirit of independence.

Known as "the island of beauty," Corsica is famous for its varied landscape, including mountains and dramatic ravines, a large network of walking trails, spectacular beaches, and stunning coastlines. The port city of Bastia in northeastern Corsica is reachable by a five-hour boat ride or a 30-minute flight from Nice. There is also a ferry that goes to Calvi on

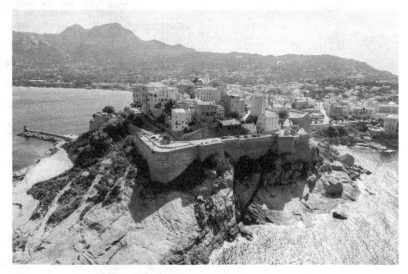

The medieval fortress in Calvi. ISTOCK.COM / NAEBLYS

the northwest coast. This picturesque port boasts that it is the birthplace of Christopher Columbus.

It is well worth taking a week to visit the entire island and fully appreciate all that it offers in terms of scenery, food, wine, culture, and music. We loved taking our niece and her husband on one of our trips to Corsica and were thrilled to see how much the experience meant to them. They returned to the U.S. with many souvenirs of Nice and Corsica.

In addition to enjoying time in Sicily, the largest island in the Mediterranean, we have visited Sardinia, also part of Italy, and the second largest Mediterranean island. Located only seven miles from the southern tip of Corsica, it has a rich history and culture along with pristine water, sandy beaches, and a rugged landscape. One of Sardinia's landmarks is its Bronze Age stone ruins.

While on a Mediterranean cruise in 2006, we made a brief visit to Crete, an island of 3,200 square miles, which has been occupied for over 130,000 years, with remnants of many civilizations. It became part of Greece in 1913. One of the lovely features of Crete is the huge mountain range that traverses the island.

On the same trip, our ship stopped at Malta, a much smaller island (96 square miles) located between Italy and Libya. We docked in the beautiful Grand Harbour, which was built in the Roman era and toured the ancient city of Valletta, the capital of this independent nation. While there, we were able to uncover some of the mysteries of the Knights of Malta, a Catholic lay religious order founded in the 11th century. We had lunch with a Maltese journalist friend who showed us some of the lovely countryside.

The most beautiful Greek island we visited is Santorini, which is in the southern Aegean Sea, southeast of the mainland of Greece. Like everyone who has been to Santorini, we were enchanted by the whitewashed, blue domed houses perched on top of high cliffs. We had magnificent views of the sea and the lava stone beaches far below.

Ancient treasures: On the Greek mainland, we explored the extraordinary archeological sites in Athens and in other areas. We also passed through the Corinth Canal, which divides the Peloponnese and the mainland of Greece, marveling at the huge rock cliffs on each side that rise almost 300

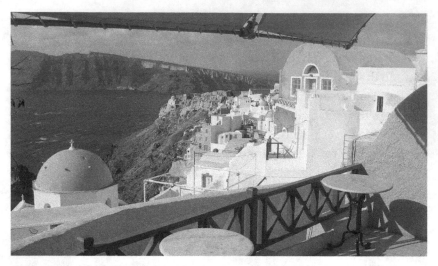

Dramatic views from Santorini, 2006

feet above the water. Although it is only four miles long and 75 feet wide, the canal was quite an architectural feat to build. The initial construction started in the first century A.D., but it was never completed. It was finally inaugurated in 1893.

Turkey is another country with a rich history and culture. Along with previous trips to see the major landmarks in Istanbul, Ankara, and surrounding areas, on the cruise we were fortunate to visit parts of the Turkish Riviera. The most spectacular stop was in Ephesus, which served as an important center of civilization beginning in the 4th century B.C. I was amazed to learn that women were granted equal rights as men at that time. We toured the Temple of Artemis, one of the Seven Wonders of the Ancient World, as well as other stunning sites nearby, including the Marble Road, the Commercial Agora, the Roman Baths, and the Celsus Library built in 117 A.D. We were treated to a dinner in front of this architectural marvel, one of the few of its kind from the Roman era. It reportedly housed 12,000 scrolls.

We also walked through the ruins of a huge amphitheater dating from the Hellenistic period. This marble structure was originally 475 feet wide and almost 100 feet tall, with room for 24,000 spectators. Before our cruise ship left Turkey, we stopped at a local bazaar to buy several small carpets for our house in Nice as a souvenir of this fascinating tour of the

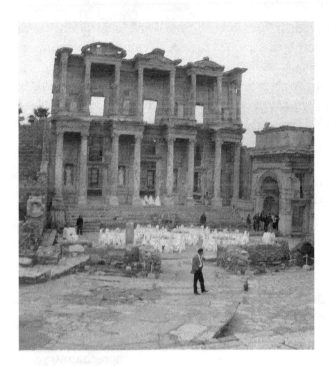

Our unforgettable evening at the Celsus Library in Ephesus, 2006

Mediterranean. Our one regret was not being able to visit historical sites near Tripoli, Libya, where we were refused entry.

Some of the most rewarding experiences of my career took place along the Mediterranean Sea's southern border, in Morocco, Tunisia, and Egypt. Terry and I have also explored the beautiful western Mediterranean coastlines of southern France and Spain.

Other Travels

Early in our marriage we did quite a bit of travelling together as well as separately for our jobs.

Exploring Terry's roots: In the mid-to-late 70s, before Terry's father (Walter Maguire) died, we accompanied his father and stepmother on several trips, including to Ireland and France. In Ireland, we found the house where Terry's paternal grandfather was raised before emigrating at age 20 to the U.S. In France, we met Maguire cousins from Ireland who were visiting Brittany at the time. We saw other Irish relatives in Normandy. They were Catholic nuns in their 90s who had been living and working there from the time they were teenagers. These were all emotional encounters.

After Terry did a lot of research and submitted his application, he was able to register his birthright Irish citizenship while maintaining his U.S. nationality. Several years later, I became a citizen, too, as his spouse. Since then, the rules have become more stringent. I would have to live in Ireland for three years before qualifying for dual citizenship.

The Pacific and Southeast Asia: We also travelled to the Pacific and Far East, stopping to see the islands of French Polynesia, which my father-in-law had visited in the early 1930s when he was under the employment of Commodore Vanderbilt and travelling on his ship around the world. The specimens he collected are on display at the Vanderbilt Museum on Long Island. We had a wonderful time visiting the stunning islands of Tahiti, Moorea, and Bora Bora. Afterwards, we moved on to the lesser-known island of Raiatea where the Vanderbilt ship had docked for a couple of weeks and young Walter Maguire became friends with a local woman. We were able to arrange for the two of them to meet again more than 40 years later. Terry and I were delighted to serve as French-English interpreters during this poignant reunion where they talked about their families and different lives.

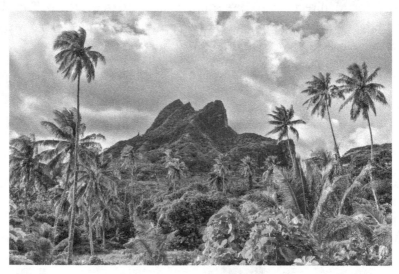

Exotic Raiatea. iStock.com / CampPhoto

On another trip, the four of us went to Hong Kong, Singapore, Indonesia, Australia, and New Zealand where we had many other adventures. One of the highlights was touring the spectacular island of Bali, with its volcanic mountains, rice paddies, and beautiful beaches along with Hindu temples that were overrun with monkeys. At one temple, I had a brief scare when a huge monkey, almost my size, jumped from an adjacent wall on top of me. Everyone around me froze. I was stunned that no one came to my rescue. Finally, I was able to free myself from the monkey's tight grip by throwing the food I was holding on the ground. This was clearly the monkey's primary interest. While the episode probably lasted only a couple of minutes, it seemed much longer to me!

Ecuador and Peru: After touring the capitals of both countries, we travelled to Cusco, Peru where we were introduced to a fascinating mixture of Spanish colonial and Incan cultures. Cusco, once the capital of the Inca Empire, is reportedly the oldest continuously inhabited city in South America. It is also located at an altitude of over 11,000 feet. After one pisco sour, the country's famous alcoholic drink, I began to feel very dizzy and quickly realized I had reached my limit.

From Cusco we made our way by train and bus to Machu Picchu, the "Lost City of the Incas," a UNESCO World Heritage Site, dating from the 15th century. It felt as though we were standing on top of the world! The views were truly breathtaking. We climbed around the ruins of the citadel, admired the temples and ceremonial baths, and watched the llamas. That evening we stayed in the small inn at the site, giving us more time to gaze at the ruins and spectacular mountain peaks and valleys in the distance.

ACCOMPANYING TERRY ON WORK-RELATED TRIPS

During the early years of my career, I took vacation time to accompany Terry on some of the Board meetings of the American Newspaper Publishers Association (now the News Media Alliance) where he served as General Counsel. This was an opportunity to get to know the major newspaper publishers at that time. I was fortunate to spend time with Punch Sulzberger of *The New York Times* and Katharine Graham of *The Washington Post*. What impressed me about these two remarkable publishers was how unassuming, warm, and engaging they were in an informal setting. We had many delightful conversations. Terry also worked with the International Federation of Newspaper Publishers (FIEJ) where I met, at annual conventions, other impressive individuals from around the world.

Through both of these organizations, Terry and I had some fascinating trips outside the U.S., including to Argentina, Japan, the U.K, France, Norway, Finland, Russia, Italy, Spain, Hungary, and the Czech Republic as well as Monaco, among other places. In Monaco, the group of 30 publishers, spouses, and staff had a private meeting at the Prince's Palace with the royal family, a tour of the underground wine cellars where precious paintings and wines were hidden during World War II, and an elegant private meal at the famous Louis XV restaurant. We were briefed by the Head of the Sixth Fleet and visited a U.S. aircraft carrier off the port of Monte Carlo, which was a floating city housing 5,000 sailors. These were just some of the adventures we shared as part of Terry's work.

GIVING TERRY A FIRST-HAND VIEW OF MY WORK

Terry accompanied me on overseas travels only a few times during my career, including the first trip we took to Africa in the early 1970s. Another unforgettable trip was to Tunisia in the 1980s. I had already arrived in Tunis and was busy with meetings. One of my Tunisian colleagues, Anwar, accompanied me to the airport to meet Terry. We waited until all the passengers had disembarked, having caught a brief glimpse of him in the line. However, we began to worry when Terry never reappeared. We learned that he was being held by airport police.

The reason why Terry was detained was that he reported his profession on his entry form as a journalist/lawyer. At that time, Tunis was hosting an important conference and the government was extremely nervous about members of the foreign press and lawyers entering the country. Fortunately, Anwar was a close friend of the head of the airport. Getting Terry released turned out to be less challenging than I feared, despite the great anxiety we all felt at the time. After this incident, Terry enjoyed meeting many of my Tunisian colleagues and accompanied me on visits to several health facilities. The most fascinating experience for Terry was seeing some USAID-supported family planning activities in rural communities south of Tunis.

Without the drama we faced in Tunisia, Terry had a chance to travel once with me during work in Morocco, Mexico, and India. We had more extraordinary experiences in each of these countries.

OUR BUCKET LIST

Our top priority is to return to our little house in Nice when travel bans are lifted, and it is safe to take a long international flight without increasing our exposure to COVID-19. In addition to spending time in our favorite places in southeastern France, we are anxious to go back to Corsica, visit friends in Italy, tour the Croatian coast, and see more of Spain and Portugal. At the end of 2020, we will celebrate our 50th anniversary—hopefully not in confinement!

While we have been fortunate to travel extensively throughout the world, together and as part of our careers, there are some special places that we would like to visit again, such as Morocco and Tunisia. We would love to return to India so that we can spend time with precious friends.

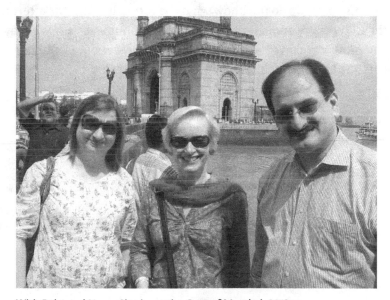

With Ruby and Nozer Sheriar at the Gate of Mumbai, 2013

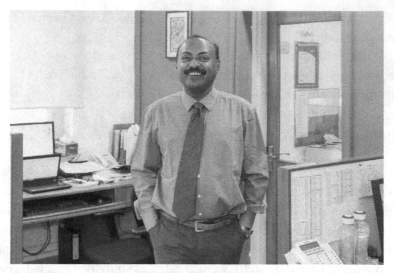

Vinoj Manning at his office in Delhi, 2017. © Ipas Development Foundation (IDF)

There are countries in Africa and Latin America as well where I would appreciate the chance to see former colleagues and relive wonderful memories.

At this point, we do not know what the future holds in the aftermath of the COVID-19 pandemic and the global economic crisis. We may be taking more virtual voyages in the future. Moreover, we will likely run out of time to check off all the items on our bucket list!

PART SIX

PERSONAL REFLECTIONS

GUIDING PRINCIPLES, LEADERSHIP, AND MENTORSHIP

19

LIVING CORE VALUES

Your beliefs become your thoughts.
Your thoughts become your words.
Your words become your actions.
Your actions become your habits.
Your habits become your values.
Your values become your destiny.
— MAHATMA GANDHI

My life and work have been deeply rooted in a set of core values—instilled by my family and inspired by the amazing people I have met and the experiences I have had around the world. People are generally motivated by a set of principles that provide a compass for life and a guide for interacting with others and getting the most out of life's experiences. Of course, these values vary from one person to another.

As the daughter and granddaughter of Episcopal ministers, I grew up going to church every Sunday and being inspired by the deep faith of my family. In my adult years, however, my church attendance dropped off. Through my travels in every continent and work with people from a wide variety of backgrounds and beliefs, I have admired the richness of different cultures and religious practices. Indeed, core values of love, compassion, kindness, forgiveness, and humility, among others, are imbedded in all major religions.

I believe that the principles I have tried to follow have enhanced my knowledge, sensitivity, and every aspect of my life. I have strived to live my core values each day. Nevertheless, there are many instances when I failed to do so. I wish I could relive those moments and respond differently.

In reflecting back over my life, each chapter has been immensely rewarding. However, like everyone, I have had some painful experiences, including the loss of loved ones and health problems. To get through these periods, I have tried to keep a positive attitude and a high level of determination as well as a longer-term perspective. I have found that maintaining a philosophy of appreciation is essential.

While I have many core values that I consider critical, I have distilled my most important ones into a list of fifteen that I have grouped into five broad categories:

- Passion – Empowerment – Perseverance

- Compassion – Love and Friendship – Gratitude

- Smiling – Enthusiasm – Optimism

- Kindness – Honesty – Humility

- Curiosity – Adventure – Continuous Learning.

I am sure that many of these have been empowering to others as well.

PASSION – EMPOWERMENT – PERSEVERANCE

~

Passion

Everyone can rise above their circumstances and achieve success if they are dedicated to and passionate about what they do.

— NELSON MANDELA

Passion appears at the top of my list of core values because it has been a driving force in my life and is pivotal to my other guiding principles. I believe that passion is essential in life and leadership.

Spending time on things we enjoy adds excitement and meaning to our lives; it enhances our personal growth, happiness, and *joie de vivre*. It makes us appreciate the richness of life. When we share our passion and enthusiasm with others, it is contagious. Everyone benefits.

In pursuing my passion, I have been able to fulfill my dreams and lead a purposeful life. I feel fortunate to have embraced a career dedicated to giving women the power to make their own reproductive decisions freely and safely. For almost five decades, I have focused on improving the health and well-being of women and children in developing countries. In the process, I hope I have helped many achieve their dreams as well.

In counselling young people, I always tell them that their top priority should be to do what excites and inspires them and allows them to learn new things each day. They should also strive to lead a life that benefits others.

~

Empowerment

There's no substitute for self-respect, banding together with other people, standing up for ourselves. Liberation does not come from outside. Power can't be given to you. The process of taking it is part of the empowerment.

— GLORIA STEINEM

Each of us needs to be empowered to follow our passion and choose our mission in life. Personal empowerment involves taking control over your life; acting in accordance with your core values; understanding your motivations, strengths, and weaknesses; and learning from your mistakes. Also key is feeling self-confident, trusting your intuition, having a good attitude, setting realistic goals for your life and work, and taking action to achieve them. Most importantly, in life and leadership, I believe that each of us has the responsibility to help others gain the tools and self-esteem they need to enhance their lives and reach their full potential.

Lifting up women and girls: There is nothing more fundamental to social and economic development and political change than the empowerment of women and girls.

In the last 45 years, I have joined with millions around the world who are fighting for these basic rights. This is an ongoing struggle and one that must be broadened and accelerated.

Over the course of my career, I have had the chance to help other women expand their own opportunities, and in turn, empower others. When women and girls stand together and support each other, great things can be accomplished. They can do more and be more. Each of us must try to be a game-changer and work with others to achieve lasting transformation in the lives of women and girls.

There have been tremendous advances in my lifetime in women's empowerment in Europe and other advanced countries, including the U.S., most recently manifested in the #MeToo movement and in the Women's Marches across the country. However, women of color and others continue to be disadvantaged and left behind. This issue must receive a much higher level of commitment and response.

In developing countries, gender inequity, in all its dimensions, remains a problem of utmost importance. All around the world, too many women are demeaned, disrespected, dismissed, disempowered, and live in abject poverty. Moreover, a shocking percentage of women and girls are victims of sexual violence, including rape as a weapon of war in conflict-torn areas. This is a global crisis!

We have a responsibility to speak for those without a voice and without a choice. We must help women and girls be heard and valued and become agents of change for themselves, their families, and their communities. This is also essential for all aspects of development, including health care, education, food security, housing, employment, water, and energy as well as addressing climate change.

How can we summon a moment of lift for human beings—and especially for women? Because when you lift up women, you lift up humanity. And how can we create a moment of lift in human hearts so that we all WANT to lift up women? Because sometimes all that's needed to lift women up is to stop pulling them down.

— MELINDA GATES,
The Moment of Lift: How Empowering Women Changes the World

The right to reproductive choice: In order for women and girls to be truly empowered, they must be able to make their own decisions about their bodies, their health, and their lives. As Professor Mahmoud Fathalla, the creator of the term "reproductive health," has highlighted: "Women are not dying because of diseases we cannot treat. They are dying because societies have yet to make the decision that their lives are worth saving." He is also famous for the phrase: "A prescription for women's health: power."

Thanks to the combined efforts of governments, non-governmental organizations, and other partners, we have seen over the past 50 years substantial increases in the availability of family planning and reproductive health care in each region. Indeed, every organization working on this issue can offer powerful testimonials from women and girls who are extremely grateful for the information, training, and services they have received and the chance to live to their full potential.

Nevertheless, according to a recent UNFPA survey, 57% of women around the world still lack the ability to make their own reproductive decisions. This is a shocking statistic when it involves a basic human right and one that is fundamental to the welfare of women and societies. Moreover, these rights are always at much greater risk during epidemics and other disasters.

~

Perseverance

You may encounter many defeats, but you must not be defeated. In fact, it may be necessary to encounter the defeats, so you know who you are, what you can rise from, how you can still come out of it.

— MAYA ANGELOU

Commitment, self-reliance, hard work, and self-discipline along with perseverance have been fundamental principles for me. These values have helped me, and millions of others, create new possibilities to make a difference. Whenever I face tough tasks, I try to break each big task into a series of smaller and manageable ones. I have found it helpful as well to look at every challenge as an opportunity, no matter how daunting the task. And I have been willing to devote whatever time and energy was necessary to get the job done. I have always been eager to engage in new tasks, be inventive, and innovate—sometimes succeeding and sometimes not—knowing that each experience will provide valuable lessons.

I believe that success in life and leadership comes with vision, passion, determination, courage, ingenuity, and never giving up. This spirit was captured in a message written in chalk on the sidewalk near our house during the coronavirus outbreak: "You can do the impossible."

The global COVID-19 pandemic has called on each of us to step up and be resilient. Making a special effort to help others is crucial in the war against this invisible enemy and in global emergencies in the future. We will persevere and advance together, with hope and strength.

It is also imperative that we accelerate the fight for social justice around the world. After 400 years of racial injustice in the U.S. and the brutal murders of innocent black men, women, and children by police officers, we must put maximum pressure on those in power to achieve real and lasting change. We must do this to honor George Floyd and all those who preceded and followed him. We must no longer tolerate the glaring inequities and inequality in the U.S. and worldwide.

COMPASSION – LOVE AND FRIENDSHIP – GRATITUDE

Compassion

I feel the capacity to care is the thing which gives life its deepest significance.

— PABLO CASALS

With my family as role models from a young age, I have always believed that listening and acting with compassion is a critical core value. Compassion means understanding and caring about what others are going through since we have all experienced—to different degrees—loss, suffering, ill health, pain, loneliness, humiliation, and fear. Showing compassion towards others also enhances our own well-being. It is a source of continuous learning, improvement, and reward.

I have been moved and inspired by so many compassionate people with whom I have worked over a 50-year period, especially the different levels of frontline health care providers I have met in Africa, Asia, and Latin America. A great many of these extraordinary people are women.

During 2020, we have experienced a period of tremendous fear, grief, and uncertainty. It is shocking and very painful to see human suffering and economic disaster of such unimaginable dimensions. The number of people impacted by the loss of loved ones and livelihoods, as well as by loneliness and confinement, is staggering and continues to grow around the world. The novel coronavirus outbreak is the greatest global crisis we have faced since World War II. And yet we are uplifted by the extraordinary compassion of health professionals, first responders, and other essential workers who are risking their lives to save those of others. Joining this outpouring of compassion are people of every age, race, ethnicity, gender, sexual orientation, socio-economic status, discipline, religion, and ideology.

Empathy is an extension of compassion when you can relate to the experience, loss, and pain of another and connect with them with your heart.

Learning to stand in somebody else's shoes, to see through their
eyes, that's how peace begins. And it's up to you to make that happen.
Empathy is a quality of character that can change the world.

— BARACK OBAMA

Since the coronavirus knows no boundaries, this pandemic is increasing
our empathy as individuals and as a global community. Another critical
cause for national and international solidarity is the struggle for racial
equality and social justice. We must all march forward under the banner
"Black Lives Matter" and turn this message into societal transformation.

~

Love and Friendship

What is a friend? A single soul dwelling in two bodies.

— ARISTOTLE

Love and friendship are life's greatest gifts. They entail putting others
first, listening to each other, caring about each other, comforting and
helping each other during good and difficult times, respecting each other,
learning from each other, forgiving each other, encouraging each other,
providing advice without judgment, and being honest. As partners and
friends, we also bring out the best in each other and serve as sources of
inspiration.

I am blessed to have wonderful friends from every stage of my life—
from Terry and my family to many other precious people, including former colleagues and fellow Board members. I appreciate all the dedicated
and dynamic individuals I have met in my travels along with partners and
allies from the international reproductive health and rights community.
These friendships have brought much joy and happiness and have been a
major part of my life. It means a lot to stay in touch via email, text, phone,
and social media. I especially like seeing friends on Skype, FaceTime,
What's App, or Zoom.

It is important during emergencies like the COVID-19 pandemic to reach out to loved ones, neighbors, and those in greatest need to provide support, from a distance. There is nothing more critical than love and friendship during a time of enormous upheaval in our daily lives.

~

Gratitude

Gratitude is not only the greatest of virtues, but the parent of all the others.

— CICERO

I am grateful to all the people who have helped me, inspired me, and taught me important lessons. My life has also been enriched by the awesome experiences I have had in countries around the world.

I believe that a person can never express too much appreciation for the small as well as the big moments in life. When we show gratitude to others, we not only make them happy, but it warms our soul as well.

I like to convey thanks in different ways—face to face, in an email or text, a handwritten note, or an ecard. In addition to the daily opportunities to make others feel good, I try to send birthday wishes to those who are special in my life. There is also Thanksgiving Day along with other important days during the year that provide perfect moments to send personal appreciation to others. Giving little gifts when you visit a friend is something I learned at a young age from my mother.

Each day, if possible, I try to provide a warm greeting, encouragement, or a compliment to at least one person. It may be someone I haven't been in contact for a while, or it may be a family member or friend with whom I talk on a regular basis. I do it sincerely without expecting anything in return. If I can help brighten someone's day, I feel content. Unfortunately, there never seems to be enough time to do all that you would like to do to thank the many people you love and admire. I have some regrets about not conveying my full gratitude to teachers and others before they died. One of my high priorities is to continue to express appreciation to all who are precious to me and who have been part of my journey.

During the coronavirus pandemic, we are especially thankful for the people who are working to save and protect lives and for those who are addressing the massive levels of unemployment and suffering. Journalists who are keeping us updated on the latest developments also deserve our praise.

SMILING – ENTHUSIASM – OPTIMISM

Smiling

Your smile is your logo, your personality is your business card, how you leave others feeling after having an experience with you becomes your trademark.

— JAY DANZIE

Interacting with others almost always makes me smile. This is a natural reflex for me. The only time in my life when I tried to refrain from smiling as much was when I wore braces on my front teeth for a couple of years as a teenager. When the braces were removed, my smiles became even bigger.

Of course, in periods of great stress, loss, or pain, smiling may be more difficult, but it is still important. For over 40 years, I have enjoyed reading an inspirational poem embossed on a plaque in my study entitled "A Smile."

Being affectionate and hugging is a trait I inherited from my mother, and she and I exchanged a lot of hugs over the years. This was reinforced during my time living in France and Italy as well as working and travelling extensively in Latin America and Africa where hugging is common among family and friends. However, not everyone wants to be hugged, and it is important to respect each person's space even among friends. Moreover, during a pandemic, we are limited to exchanging virtual hugs.

For those who like to be hugged:

. . . A hug communicates support, security, affection, unity, and belonging. A hug shows compassion. A hug brings delight. A hug charms the senses. A hug touches the soul.

— BOB STOESS

Smiling and hugging are often accompanied by laughter, which feels great as well.

When we laugh together, wonderful bonds of caring are forged.
— Alison Stormwolf

 Smiling, hugs, and laughter—even from a distance—are all easy yet powerful acts. All take only a moment and give a lot in return. They improve our relationships, boost our spirits, and enhance our mental and physical well-being. We should all take these simple steps every day, especially during difficult times.

 Our new reality of social distancing is challenging, but we must do everything possible to retain our connections to others. While schools were closed, my niece sent a video to her autistic students with the following message:

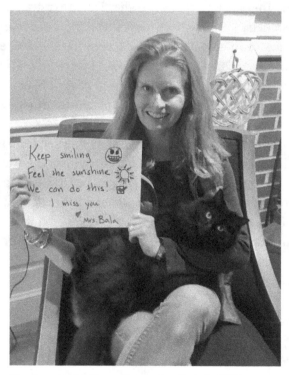

My niece, *la otra Liz*, smiling and optimistic, 2020

~

Enthusiasm

Enthusiasm is excitement with inspiration, motivation, and a pinch of creativity.

— ROBERT FOSTER BENNETT

Enthusiasm and excitement are engines that fuel our life and work. We get excited when we spend time with loved ones, meet new people, experience new ideas and places, celebrate good news and accomplishments, and are inspired by innovations. Enthusiasm can sustain us through big tasks and challenges. It helps us advance towards our goals. Sharing enthusiasm and excitement with loved ones and close friends is important. However, there are times when people like me become overly passionate and need to be careful not to interrupt others during a lively conversation. I know that I have been guilty of this!

During this tough period when we do not know what lies ahead, we must make a special effort not to lose these important qualities.

~

Optimism

Optimism is the faith that leads to achievement. Nothing can be done without hope and confidence.

— HELEN KELLER

Among my fundamental values are optimism and positivity. They have helped me through some tough moments and enabled me to lead a happy and fulfilling life. As someone who has always viewed "the glass half full," I believe this characteristic has been very motivating for me and spurred my efforts to make meaningful contributions in life. I hope that my positivity has added bright spots in the lives of others.

There are periods when optimism must be tempered with realism, along with faith in the power of the human spirit and the enormous collective difference that people can make. This is certainly the case during local, national, and global disasters. Retaining a level of optimism can help us be more resilient as we deal with the stress and uncertainty from the COVID-19 pandemic and as we fight for social and economic justice.

Kindness – Honesty – Humility

Transcending other values are kindness, honesty, integrity, and humility. These principles were engrained in me in my childhood, and I have tried to practice them in the best way I can.

~

Kindness

Kindness is more than deeds. It is an attitude, an expression, a look, a touch. It is anything that lifts another person.

—Plato

Being kind and generous does indeed lift people's spirits. Even small acts, such as giving a small gift or conveying appreciation, can have a large impact.

I have witnessed countless acts of kindness by family, friends, colleagues, acquaintances, and strangers. These gestures always inspire me to do more and be more. During my travels throughout the developing world, I have been overwhelmed by the warmth and kindness of people whom I have never met before, including those living in extreme poverty. They have offered me something to drink or eat even though they may not know when they will have their next meal.

Kindness has been on heightened display around the world during the COVID-19 crisis. Every day we see countless examples of selflessness and generosity. We hear so many stories of people volunteering to make masks and other personal protective equipment, donate blood and plasma, and deliver food and other supplies. We are moved when we see on TV individuals clapping, singing, and giving thanks to doctors, nurses, and other essential workers. We smile when we read messages of hope and perseverance written in chalk on sidewalks. We are comforted by the stories of all who are checking in regularly by phone or FaceTime with people living alone or in nursing homes. And our spirits are boosted when artists and musicians share their work with us on social media.

In a burst of kindness and creativity, the rock musician Bon Jovi shared on social media in late March 2020 a video and song to cheer and support people during this unprecedented period. In the chorus, he sings, "When you can't do what you do, you do what you can . . . ." Bon Jovi invited fans to share their stories so that he can incorporate as many as feasible into the lyrics of this evolving coronavirus song. Willie Nelson, singing with his sons, did a rendition of his famous song "On the road again" offering hope of what people can look forward to as they emerge from confinement. These are just two examples of a long list of musicians trying to lift our spirits.

> *Kindness currency is absolutely free, and anyone can give it.*
> — LADY GAGA

We were treated, in mid-April, to a virtual eight-hour music and cultural extravaganza, "One World: Together at Home," an initiative curated by Lady Gaga working with Global Citizen. Hosted by Jimmy Kimmel, Jimmy Fallon, and Stephen Colbert, the program featured artists from around the world, including Stevie Wonder with "Lean on me", Jennifer Lopez with her rendition of "People", John Legend and Sam Smith performing "Stand by Me", and Taylor Swift with "Soon You'll Get Better." For the finale, Céline Dion and Andrea Bocelli sang "The Prayer", joined by Lady Gaga, John Legend, and pianist Lang Lang. There were many other artists who participated in this epic event. The concert was live streamed on multiple global platforms, honoring frontline health professionals and other key workers. The goal was to provide funding for essential supplies through multiple organizations as well as to support WHO's COVID-19 Solidarity Response Fund. The concert raised almost $128 million for these relief efforts in addition to the $50 million already pledged.

In late May, I received a link to a video from Vinoj Manning, CEO of IDF in India, which supports women's access to essential reproductive health care. It was an impressive expression of team bonding during a stressful time. In the video, 159 quarantined staff, working from home in 42 locations in 12 states, sang in their local languages "We shall overcome." I was moved to tears when I watched it and was uplifted by such a powerful message of hope and courage.

For all who can provide financial support, there are many outstanding organizations and groups helping to meet the basic needs of the most vulnerable during these challenging times.

~

Honesty

We learned about honesty and integrity   that the truth matters . . . that you don't take shortcuts or play by your own set of rules . . . and success doesn't count unless you earn it fair and square.

— MICHELLE OBAMA

Being open and honest with everyone as well as living with integrity means adhering to high moral and ethical standards. Along with others, I try to follow these universal principles in my daily life, albeit sometimes imperfectly. Unfortunately, speaking the truth may not always feel good to others, but it is essential. The current public health pandemic is a compelling example of why we need our leaders to tell us the full truth.

During the height of the COVID-19 outbreak, I appreciated the daily televised press conferences by Governor Cuomo of New York. In delivering the latest update on the coronavirus, he consistently based his remarks and decisions on science and the facts and spoke with compassion. This is in sharp contrast to what we have heard from President Trump.

~

Humility

Humility is the solid foundation of all virtues.

— CONFUCIUS

My parents and grandparents provided powerful examples of respect and humility. They taught me how critical these values are in life, in the workplace, and in leadership.

Being humble means focusing on others rather than on yourself. I respect and admire friends and colleagues who have different skills and experience and welcome the opportunity to learn from and be inspired by them. Humility, unfortunately, does not seem as common as other virtues.

I always feel humble in the presence of truly great leaders who have dedicated their lives to lifting up their communities as well as those who have had an even broader impact on the welfare of their country and our global society. In the field of women's reproductive health and rights, Professor Mahmoud Fathalla is extraordinarily articulate, compassionate, and humble. Former President Barack Obama and Dr. Martin Luther King, Jr. are towering figures in U.S. and world history who, along with Presidents Carter and Lincoln, among others, exhibited these characteristics as well. Nelson Mandela will go down in history as one of the most eloquent and humble leaders of all times. There are, of course, countless others who belong on this list.

In my work in developing countries, I have also experienced true humility in the presence of women and families living in a poor village or in a large urban slum. They work so hard with so little just to exist from one day to another and are examples of great courage. This is also true of frontline health care providers who face every day demanding conditions and inadequate facilities and equipment in their efforts to save people's lives.

Curiosity – Adventure – Continuous Learning

Curiosity

Creative people are curious, flexible, persistent, and independent with a tremendous spirit of adventure and a love of play.

— Henri Matisse

I believe that living life with a high level of curiosity and using your imagination to the fullest leads to greater creativity, innovation, and impact. It is energizing and exciting to learn something new each day, to look at different ways of doing things, and to do new things. The same spark that each of us feels from being curious and innovative can impact others, too. These are opportunities we should all embrace.

We are fortunate to be surrounded and inspired by scientists, artists, and people of all disciplines who display enormous creativity and inventiveness and who contribute to advancements in our society every day. The worst of times are generally ones of enormous creativity and innovation. We are living in an unprecedented moment in our history. We must emerge from the current pandemic and the fight for equality with new, creative ways to build a global society that lifts up everyone.

Innovation is the pursuit of what can be, unburdened by what has been. And we pursue innovation not because we are bored but because we want to make things faster, more efficient, more effective, more accurate.

— Kamala Harris,
The Truths We Hold: An American Journey

~

Fun and Adventure

Life is not measured by the number of breaths you take but by the moments that take your breath away.

— MAYA ANGELOU

Dreaming, exploration, discovery, adventure, and fun are fundamental parts of life. Everyone deserves these chances for personal enjoyment and growth. My advice is to record the most memorable experiences in real time. This is something I wish I had done systematically during my life.

I am grateful for all the moments I have had throughout my life for exploration and discovery. In addition to living in England, France, and Italy, I have been fortunate to travel to 85 countries, including visiting and/or working in 40 countries in Africa, Asia, and Latin America. Many of these countries I have visited multiple times, sometimes for extended periods. All these trips have given me a rich perspective on life—the opportunity to experience and value other cultures and traditions, admire historical landmarks and beautiful scenery, and appreciate local cuisine, art, handicrafts, literature, music, dance, and religious practices.

Most of all, I have loved the thrill of meeting and learning from interesting people. A number of these individuals have become cherished friends. This has certainly been the most satisfying and uplifting part of my life.

~

Continuous Learning

Live as if you were to die tomorrow. Learn as if you were to live forever.

— MAHATMA GANDHI

We know that learning is limitless and that reaching your full potential is a lifelong exercise. For me, this includes learning from my mistakes and making improvements as well as trying to emulate the best in others.

There are always new adventures, discoveries, and rewarding experiences ahead.

During periods of confinement and physical distancing, we can try to read more and benefit from online learning, ranging from exercises and healthy eating to studying another language, engaging in crafts, participating in webinars, and exploring new topics and places. We can also appreciate virtual performances of orchestras, tour museum exhibits online, watch movies and plays, and admire nature's wonders around the world. I was pleased that the city of Nice has a site entitled "Cultivez-Vous," offering links for people to enjoy "moments of curiosity, sharing, and emotion."

I look forward to all the opportunities to learn and do more in the years ahead, hopefully not in confinement. I also want to remain engaged in helping others advance and achieve their dreams.

20

THOUGHTS ON LEADERSHIP

The leaders whom I have known personally and admire greatly are pioneers and visionaries. They are eloquent, passionate, and courageous. Through their inspirational leadership, and in partnership with others, they have helped advance women's reproductive health and rights around the world. They have left lasting legacies and motivated new generations of leaders. A number of these giants have also exhibited tremendous warmth, kindness, generosity, and humility despite their world-renowned status.

There are many other leaders in the reproductive health and rights field who are less well known but who are making a real difference in advancing the work and impact of their organizations. I continue to be excited by talented leaders of all ages and disciplines. I also have high expectations for the youngest generation of leaders.

In this chapter, I reflect on some of the writings on leadership, general responsibilities of leaders, personal leadership qualities, performance during a crisis, and the continuing gender and wage gap.

BOOKS ON LEADERSHIP

The market is flooded with books on leadership, discussing core principles, theories, and models along with strategies for leading organizations to greatness and enhancing personal leadership skills. There are also a huge number of books on related topics, such as organizational development, teamwork, management practices, governance, career success, growth mindset, and professional self-help and advancement, to mention a few.

Until recently, the vast majority of books on leadership have been written by men, reflecting the tremendous gender imbalance at the highest levels of companies and organizations. Also, most of these books focus on the business sector and a much smaller percentage on how to be an effective leader in the public and non-profit sectors. Nevertheless, there are important principles that apply to all sectors.

One of the oldest and most widely read books on leadership is *How to Win Friends and Influence People* written by Dale Carnegie in 1936 which addresses, among other things, networking and relationship-building skills. There have been subsequent editions, including one focused on the digital age. In 1987, Jim Kouzes and Barry Posner wrote *The Leadership Challenge: How to Get Extraordinary Things Done in Organizations*. They reflect on what makes a great leader, including how to inspire a shared vision, empower your team, and challenge the process. This award-winning book, available in 22 languages, was the first of many books by these two authors, including *The Truth about Leadership*, published in 2010. Based on 30 years of research, it highlights the key characteristics of trust, credibility, and ethics, among other core principles. The seventh edition of *The Leadership Challenge* was published in 2017.

In 1989, Stephen Covey wrote the best seller *The 7 Habits of Highly Effective People*, in which he highlights the importance of being pro-active, "thinking win-win," positive teamwork, and continuous improvement. Many of these themes are echoed in subsequent books by Covey and other experts on leadership.

One of the most prolific writers on leadership is John Maxwell whose books span the period 1993 to 2020, with likely more to come. He covers topics such as the most critical leadership qualities, how to learn from your mistakes, and the limitless capacity of leaders. His latest book is entitled *The Leader's Greatest Return: Attracting, Developing, and Multiplying Leaders*.

Another writer is Seth Godin whose books on leadership include *Tribes: We Need You to Lead Us* (2008). There is also Daniel Pink's thought-provoking book *The Surprising Truth about What Motivates Us* (2009) which comments on the elements of people's true motivation—autonomy, mastery, and purpose. Another comprehensive book on leadership, published in 2013, is *12 Disciplines of Leadership Excellence: How Leaders Achieve Sustainable High Performance* by Brian Tracy and Peter Chee.

Women entrepreneurs are increasingly sharing their advice on life and leadership, adding critical perspectives. Selena Rezvani's *The Next Generation of Women Leaders: What You Need to Lead but Won't Learn in Business School*, published in 2009, contains inspirational stories of 30 of the most successful women in high-ranking positions in their respective areas. In 2012, Rezvani's book *Pushback: How Smart Women Ask—and Stand Up—for What They Want* focuses on negotiating skills and other key issues. Sheryl Sandberg, in her 2013 book *Lean In: Women, Work, and the Will to Lead*, recounts her own experiences, her successes and mistakes, and provides guidance on how best to act and achieve your goals.

How Remarkable Women Lead: The Breakthrough Model for Work and Life (2009) by Geoffrey Lewis, Joanna Barsh, and Susie Cranston is an engaging and insightful book, drawing on interviews with successful women around the world and coming up with a formula for success called "Centered Leadership." Another interesting book is *Act Like a Leader, Think Like a Leader* by Herminia Ibarra (2015) where she offers advice on how to make changes in your job, networks, and yourself. There are many other women writing about leadership, including Brené Brown whose book *Dare to Lead: Brave Work. Tough Conversations. Whole Hearts* (2018) is based on interviews with leaders from all sectors. There is a particularly insightful discussion of courage and what the author characterizes as its four key skill sets: "rumbling with vulnerability, living into our values, braving trust, and learning to rise."

Although there are currently a relatively small number of books geared for young leaders, this number will also grow, as will the blogs that offer helpful insights and guidance. Sheryl Sandberg has written a follow-on book to *Lean In*, entitled *Lean In for Graduates* where she provides tips for young people on writing résumés; preparing well for interviews; negotiating tactics; converting long-term goals into manageable steps; expanding self-confidence, skills and experience; trusting intuition; building a support network; and how to balance a career and family life.

While there are valuable lessons and advice for women and young leaders in all these books, they focus primarily on careers in the corporate sector. It is unfortunate, in my opinion, that there are not more books profiling women leaders in the global not-for-profit sector, who can share lessons and recommendations for those who would like to work, or who have already chosen careers in international development.

RESPONSIBILITIES OF LEADERS

On an organizational level, whether in business or in the non-profit sector, all leaders must ensure that there is a clear vision and mission, comprehensive strategy and action plans, sound structure, core values, effective and efficient systems, and accountability. They must mobilize the necessary human and financial resources; engage the full commitment, energy, and talents of the staff; create a dynamic and rewarding workplace; make wise decisions; and deliver strong results.

From the perspective of a former CEO of a large international non-profit and a former senior U.S. government official, there are other important lessons that I, and many others, have learned. These include: recruit, mentor, retain, and reward outstanding staff; and prioritize having a diverse, multi-disciplinary, and multi-generational team with members who complement each other well in terms of skills, experience, personality, and perspectives. Other lessons are: tap the talents of the entire team; multi-task effectively; decentralize and streamline decision-making; and set clear roles, responsibilities, and expectations.

Leaders must be effective change agents. They need to set the example and encourage staff to be bold, think outside the box, and come up with new ideas and approaches. Prudent risk-taking should be encouraged along with the understanding that not every initiative is successful but will always be instructive. Continuous innovation is key to sustained change and impact while acknowledging that there will be failures along the way. Every program should be results oriented and evidence based. There must be a strong monitoring and evaluation system and regular assessments to see what is working well and what is not. Appropriate adjustments must be made and new strategies adopted whenever needed. Regular reports on progress to date—along with "a look ahead"—are also critical. Accomplishments, big and small, should be celebrated, while always maintaining a longer-term perspective. Strategic partnerships are essential to achieving a broader impact.

CEOs must ensure for their donors and stakeholders good value for investment. They must also maintain a strong relationship with their Board of Directors, work effectively with partners, and be compelling representatives of the mission and work of their respective organizations.

PERSONAL LEADERSHIP QUALITIES

Great leadership usually starts with a willing heart, a positive attitude, and a desire to make a difference.

— MAC ANDERSON

There is no perfect leadership type. Each of us has strengths, weaknesses, and vulnerabilities. In the words of Brené Brown, the best-selling author, "Vulnerability is not knowing victory or defeat, it's understanding the necessity of both; it's engaging. It's being all in."

While each leader is different, I believe that there are some common characteristics that great leaders share. Many effective leaders have natural leadership abilities. Others need to spend time building these skills. All leaders benefit from an ongoing effort to improve their ability to communicate effectively and inspire action as well as enhance their expertise, experience, and impact.

There are dimensions of leaders, especially in a non-profit organization, that are pivotal, in my opinion—their core values and personal characteristics, including their emotional intelligence. The qualities that I believe are key include ones discussed in the last chapter: passion; empowerment; perseverance; compassion and empathy; expressing appreciation; exchanging smiles and laughter; sharing enthusiasm and positivity; displaying genuine kindness and generosity; and showing honesty and integrity, respect, humility, curiosity, and creativity. It is also important to have fun!

Leaders should check their egos at the front door and shine the spotlight on the staff instead, recognizing that the real strength of an organization lies in the commitment and contributions of the members of their team. CEOs must inspire, motivate, energize, empower, and enable staff to reach their full potential. They should be self-confident and collaborative, approaching everything and everybody with an open heart and mind. Leaders should have excellent interpersonal skills and do everything possible to provide a warm, open, respectful, vibrant, and satisfying work environment where everyone's ideas are encouraged and valued. There should be an emphasis on balancing advocacy with inquiry and the need to clarify assumptions, beliefs, and feelings.

Leaders must always be flexible and adaptable, have a good sense of humor, and remain calm during challenging periods. They must also be tenacious, resilient, hopeful, and never give up. Especially during periods of significant change, leaders need to ensure an environment of trust and provide strong support to the staff. They must always be prepared to make short and long-term decisions as well as mistakes along the way.

Leaders should work hard at being their best, while acknowledging their weaknesses, and set an example of excellence and optimism for the rest of the team. Everyone should have the ability to contribute to the success of the organization. CEOs should embrace different viewpoints and deal effectively with criticism as well as recommendations for change. This is important but not always easy.

I believe in delivering plenty of positive reinforcement and thanking team members regularly for their contributions. At the same time, CEOs must provide constructive feedback and hold staff accountable for delivering results. When necessary, they must take corrective action.

Staff should be encouraged to maintain a good work-life balance and be supported during times of ill health, a family emergency, or the loss of a loved one. Leaders, like staff, should have 360-degree annual reviews and a philosophy of continuous improvement, using coaches as needed and taking full advantage of skills training and enhancement. Having an "open-door" policy is essential, in my opinion, along with encouraging staff to share concerns and suggestions. I recommend having confidential suggestion boxes and annual organizational climate surveys.

Another pivotal quality of leaders is that they must be empathetic listeners, and excellent communicators, using all forms of communication regularly. There can never be too much listening or too much communicating.

*People will always notice something about you. It might be the way
you walk or the way your talk, or just simply your personality. Live
each day in the way you want to be remembered. Live in such a way
that people will be inspired by those unique qualities that you have
and strive to live better lives for themselves.*

— AMAKA IMANI NKOSAZANA

LEADERSHIP DURING CHALLENGING TIMES

The true test of leadership is how well you function in a crisis.

— BRIAN TRACY

During the COVID-19 pandemic and its aftermath, my heart goes out
to all leaders—in federal, state, and local governments, as well as in the
non-profit and for-profit sectors, in the U.S. and around the world. While
leaders always work with different scenarios— planning for the worst and
hoping for the best—many are not well trained in crisis management. No
one—especially not the Trump White House—was prepared to deal with
an emergency of this magnitude and its myriad implications. Few people
focused on imagining the unimaginable.

Along with the extraordinary efforts of health care providers and first
responders, leaders everywhere are dealing with an incredible level of
stress during this period. They worry about the health and well-being
of their loved ones and staff as well as the status and future of the work
they oversee. Leaders, together with their staff, are coping with working
remotely as well as reconfiguring workplaces and schedules to ensure
social distancing. An overriding concern is how to cover expenses and
address people's basic needs during an indefinite period.

There are, of course, significant differences between government programs, non-profit organizations, and big and small businesses. However,
most are dealing with huge financial difficulties and the need to lay off
staff and cut vital programs. We are living in a time when the continued
existence of many organizations and businesses is uncertain.

Leaders never handle a crisis alone. They must tap all the necessary
skills and expertise they can access to develop and execute the most ef-

fective plans and make needed adjustments along the way. It is during periods of crisis that the true character of leaders is on display.

Despite advance warnings of this public health emergency, President Trump and his Administration did not take early and decisive action to prepare for, contain, and mitigate this pandemic. We witnessed an appalling lack of advance planning and inexcusable shortfalls in testing and contact tracing. Because President Trump refused to order U.S. industries to produce all that was needed to respond to the COVID-19 outbreak, there have been prolonged delays in securing sufficient test kits, critical protective gear, and other medical equipment and supplies. We have also been subjected to constant false, misleading, and conflicting statements by the president. Denying any responsibility for this national tragedy, President Trump has clearly been more concerned about his personal interests than the well-being of the American people. As the historian Jon Meacham commented recently, "The president likes to say that he is a hero but does nothing heroic."

Unlike other countries, the U.S. did not develop a comprehensive, strategic, and well-coordinated nationwide plan. Instead, what we have seen from President Trump are ad hoc and misguided decisions that have often hindered effective measures at the state and local level. Moreover, the president has refused to wear a mask and to call on Americans to protect each other's lives. Rather than unite the country in a time of crisis, he has continued to serve as a divisive force. The colossal failure of national leadership has had a devastating impact in terms of the number of lives and livelihoods lost, especially among people of color and the elderly population. In contrast to the huge shortcomings and chaos of the Trump White House, there are many other leaders who have impressed us with their dedication and performance during COVID-19 as well as during the protests against police violence, systemic racism, and injustice.

We count on our leaders to tell us the truth, no matter how painful it may be, because this is what results in trust and hope. In a time of tremendous loss and anxiety, we expect leaders to show great courage and vision as well as compassion and empathy. Their highest priority must always be on saving and protecting people's lives. We want our leaders to rely heavily on experts, make evidence-based decisions, convey consistent messages, and update us constantly with the facts. They must reassure us that all the necessary measures are being taken, that we will get through these ordeals, and that we will move forward together. We must hold our leaders accountable for their actions and results.

We are deeply grateful for the exceptional heroism of all the essential workers and the generous acts of individuals throughout the U.S. and around the world in response to the novel coronavirus outbreak. Let us hope that all leaders fulfill their responsibilities to the best of their abilities and live their "finest hour." Most importantly, we must learn from this global pandemic and other challenges we face. We must ensure that everything possible is being done to restore people's well-being and that aggressive action is being taken to mitigate the impact of current and future crises. In the meantime, we must deal with tremendous and prolonged suffering, a severe economic downturn, and a very lengthy recovery around the world.

Closing the Gender and Wage Gap

In good times and bad, women around the world have demonstrated that they can be truly transformational leaders. And yet, as noted earlier, women are still greatly underrepresented at the leadership level compared to men. This is true in government, the corporate world, and the non-profit sector. What is particularly glaring and concerning is that women of color and younger women are substantially disadvantaged in terms of filling senior leadership positions.

Globally, there is still a long way to go before gender equity and full diversity in leadership are achieved. This applies to working women of all ages, ethnicities, and backgrounds. According to the International Labour Organization, there are only six countries in the world where women and men enjoy equal legal work rights.

The issue of equal pay for equal work was headline news around the world during the fourth World Cup victory in July 2019 of the U.S. Women's National Soccer Team. In the U.S., women who have full-time employment only earn, on average, 80% of what men earn for the same job. This gap is substantially greater between women of color and white men, and at higher levels of employment, especially at the executive level.

An increasing number of studies and books are focusing on these issues. A comprehensive study conducted by Glassdoor in 2019 states that, at current rates, the gender pay gap will not be closed until 2070—a sobering conclusion! Among the books that address this critical topic are: *Ask For It: How Women Can Use the Power of Negotiation to Get What They Really Want* by Linda Babcock and Sara Laschever (2008). In an updated version of an earlier book, Mika Brzezinski wrote *Know Your Value: Women, Money, and Getting What You're Worth* (2018). Both books, which focus on the corporate sector in the U.S., have tips on how women can become better recognized and successful as well as compensated fairly.

Let's hope that the commitment by Melinda Gates in October 2019 to contribute $1 billion over the next 10 years to expanding women's equality, power, and influence in the U.S. will provide a strong impetus for other very wealthy philanthropists around the world to take similar action.

Women's role in leadership and equal pay for equal work are issues that deserve much higher priority. We must see meaningful change. We cannot accept the current situation!

21

EMPOWERING THE
NEXT GENERATIONS

A mentor is someone who allows you to see the hope inside yourself.
— OPRAH WINFREY

We have all been fortunate to have mentors during our lives. I am especially grateful for the privilege of working with two such extraordinary global leaders in the SRHR field as Professor Fred Sai of Ghana and Professor Mahmoud Fathalla of Egypt. It was always inspiring to be in their presence, and I treasured our friendship over a 30-year period. Fred Sai had a remarkable life and career, dying in September 2019 at the age of 95. I continue to be in touch with Mahmoud Fathalla. These two heroes taught me important lessons in life and leadership.

I am also thankful for the many moments I shared, over this same period, with Dr. Nafis Sadik from Pakistan, another remarkable leader and the first woman to serve as Executive Director of the United Nations Population Fund. Throughout her long tenure at the UN, she was a courageous and tireless champion of women's reproductive health and rights. Ambassador Dr. Eunice Brookman-Amissah of Ghana, who served as Ipas's Vice President for Africa during my tenure, has been a powerful advocate for girls' and women's access to comprehensive abortion care in Africa and around the world.

During my career, I had exceptional colleagues at USAID and Ipas and learned a great deal from them as well as from others I met around the world. I am indebted to Dr. Nozer Sheriar, Dr. Pouru Bhiwandi, and all the

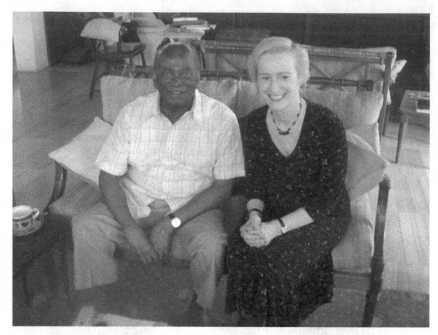

With Professor Sai at his home in Accra, 2011. BARBARA CRANE

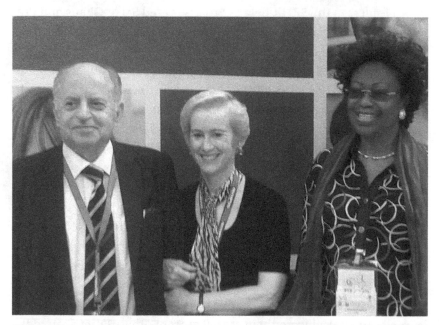

With Professor Fathalla and Dr. Brookman-Amissah at the FIGO XX World Congress in Rome, 2012

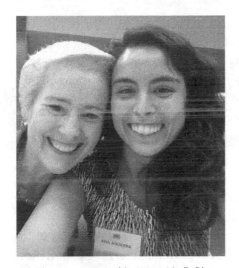

Enjoying our partnership, 2016: Liz (left) and Ana (right)

other international leaders who served on the Ipas Board. I and others benefitted greatly from their vision, insights, expertise, and compassion. Indeed, there is a long list of people who were teachers and role models for me.

Just as we admire our mentors, each of us has the responsibility to serve as a mentor to others. It is critical that we listen to, guide, support, and empower the next generations of leaders. I believe that intergenerational mentoring brings great value both to the mentor and mentee. We all have a chance to inspire and be inspired through sharing our passions, ideas, experiences, hopes, and lessons learned. My former Ipas colleague and dear friend, Ana Aguilera, and I continue to appreciate this rich exchange. And thanks to the hard work of Ana and others, I was able to mentor for the first two years after I retired young Ipas staff from each region who were supported by the Maguire Fellowship for Young Leaders.

The experience of mentoring and empowering others to reach their full potential has been immensely rewarding for me. For the past several decades, I have had the chance to mentor, on an informal basis, young people from different backgrounds and countries in Africa, Asia, and Latin America, as well as in the U.S. While these individuals cover a range of experiences, skill sets, and styles, they share many commonalities. They have all been eager to learn not just from my experience but from others within and outside their workplace. Each one has been anxious to grow personally and professionally and to improve the welfare of others.

The questions I have received from these young people have been surprisingly similar. Our discussions have focused a lot on leadership styles, confidence and relationship building, how to solicit and give feedback, surviving through good and tough times, when to switch jobs or organizations, and how to climb the leadership ladder.

I always encourage young people to look for opportunities for professional growth and new experiences every couple of years, especially early in their careers. This will help them gain additional skills, self-esteem, and perspectives. As these young people revise their CVs and apply for a new position, I have underscored the importance of highlighting their professional goals and all their relevant skills and experiences along with outlining in a cover letter how they can best contribute to the mission and work of the organization.

In addition, I advise young professionals to focus on what is most meaningful to them. They must also follow their intuition, tap their creativity, use their ingenuity, embrace the challenges and opportunities, amplify their voices, and commit to continuous improvement. Volunteering for special assignments can be a powerful learning experience. Advocating effectively for yourself and others is also paramount. Young leaders should always be prepared to demonstrate their unique value and ask for more responsibilities with commensurate compensation.

One of the questions that has surfaced is what advice I have for "introverts" who want to be great leaders. While it is unrealistic to think that an individual can make a big personality transformation, you can certainly make changes in the actions you take, such as working on listening carefully and soliciting feedback from colleagues and supervisors on what you should keep doing or modify. Learning to be an effective communicator, both orally and in writing, is also critical, along with how to motivate and empower others. No one should be afraid to ask for help or advice. Establishing a personal action plan and introducing steady, incremental improvements can make a difference.

I routinely get asked about what to do when faced with a challenge or setback. While it depends very much on the circumstance, my general response has been to keep focused on the big picture and maintain your passion, positive attitude, courage, resilience, and perseverance. In dealing with a major problem, it is always important to regroup and strategize, soliciting the ideas and skills of key members of your team and assessing optimal solutions. In the process, I have found that seeking the advice of mentors as well as using a coach or facilitator can be helpful. If there are issues around conflict management, then training and facilitation in this area are beneficial. Finally, it is critical to move forward after a setback, putting the lessons learned to good use.

Another key area is building your network of support, using both peers and mentors. For women who are working in a predominantly male environment, standing together as women and supporting each other is essential. The same is true for men in a female-dominated workplace. There are always valuable lessons to be gained from watching other leaders around you as well as reading biographies and autobiographies of people you admire.

I have been very heartened to see that the young people I have mentored have been able to follow their passion, gain beneficial skills and experience, and take on higher levels of responsibility in their chosen areas of work. As they have advanced, they have broadened their networks and used me more as a "sounding board," especially for big decisions and major life choices.

For the young leaders who are focused on empowering women and girls around the world to exercise their fundamental rights, I have urged them to do whatever they can to accelerate global action. We need to expand coalitions and networks to have a much more significant and lasting impact. No matter how difficult working on these issues may become, giving up should not be an option.

As women, we must stand up for ourselves . . . . As women, we must stand up for each other . . . . As women, we must stand up for justice for all.

— MICHELLE OBAMA

Youth activism and young leaders are vital to driving social and cultural change, including ensuring that women and girls can control their reproductive lives and their futures. I hope that increasing numbers of young people will embrace this area of work and support others in using their own voices. This work is so fundamental to helping women and girls improve their own health and the well-being of their families, gain access to a good education and job, reach their full potential, and be pivotal players in fighting for respect and justice, ending poverty, and saving our planet.

CONCLUSION

*There can be no greater gift than that of giving one's time and energy
to help others without expecting anything in return.*

— NELSON MANDELA

As I reflect on my work and life to date, I am enormously appreciative of
all that I have received—from Terry, my family, and my friends around
the world. Through my work and travels, I have met truly remarkable
people and have enjoyed many unforgettable experiences, enriching my
life beyond my wildest expectations. I hope that the reflections in *Advancing Reproductive Choice: Leading with Conviction and Compassion* will be
motivating and useful for others in their own journeys.

I feel privileged to have worked on such a core issue as helping women
and girls gain access to the comprehensive reproductive health care they
need. In collaboration with many colleagues and partners, I have had
the chance to contribute to important advances in this field. At the same
time, the unfinished agenda remains overwhelming, especially against
the backdrop of the COVID-19 pandemic. While the full impact of this
global public health crisis is still unfolding, we must not lose sight of
the imperative of ensuring that women and girls around the world can
exercise their fundamental rights and enjoy a better future. This goal *is*
attainable with the necessary political commitment and resources!

The COVID-19 pandemic has dramatically changed our lives and likely
the way we will live in the future. It is resulting in a tragedy of immense
and growing proportions in terms of the number of deaths, shattered
lives, broken health systems, and economic disasters. People around the
world are dealing with fear and loss every day. Those who are suffering
the most are the poor and most vulnerable. This is especially true for
women and girls in developing countries where hunger, disease, poverty,
and inequality are on the rise.

Recognizing that we face enormous challenges and uncertainties
ahead, each of us must focus on being the best we can be and on making
our individual contributions to improving the well-being of others. Liv-

ing our core values and staying connected to each other are more critical now than ever. Unprecedented times provide unique opportunities for positive change, creative solutions, and renewed hope. We have a chance to reimagine the future and create a better world. While dealing with COVID-19 and other crises ahead, I am counting on the next generations of leaders, particularly women, to fight for their rights, be bold and innovative, and challenge and correct inequities.

Each of us has a role to play in contributing to the goals of social justice and human rights for all individuals. This includes gender equality, empowerment, and equal access to health care, education, employment, and all life's necessities. We must continue to learn from and motivate each other. Together, we must build a more equitable and sustainable future for all members of our global society!

Let us make our future now, and let us make our dreams tomorrow's reality.

— MALALA YOUSAFZAI

ACKNOWLEDGMENTS

This book emerged out of a deep sense of gratitude, beginning with my family who imbued in me a set of core values and enabled me to grow up surrounded by love and laughter and to benefit from a good education, travel, and life-changing opportunities. I am indebted to the many friends and colleagues with whom I worked at different stages of my career, from my early experiences at Voice of America and the Population Reference Bureau to my more than two decades at USAID and 16 years at Ipas. I have also enjoyed working with talented and dedicated people from a wide array of international, regional, and national SRHR organizations, including serving as a Board member of a few of them.

I want to express my appreciation to those who have been mentors to me as well as others I have mentored over the years. I salute everyone who is continuing to advance SRHR issues at a local, national, regional, and/or global level.

This book is a tribute to health care providers who are working in challenging environments in developing countries as well as to all individuals who are trying to exercise their sexual and reproductive rights while overcoming many obstacles.

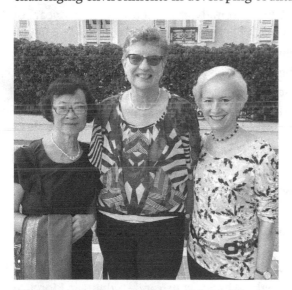

Headed to an evening concert at the Prince's Palace in Monaco, 2018: Mary, Barbara, and Liz (left to right)

As I began to write about some of my personal and professional experiences, I was encouraged by my close friends Ann Leonard and Barbara Crane to continue this project despite doubts I had about whether this was a worthwhile endeavor.

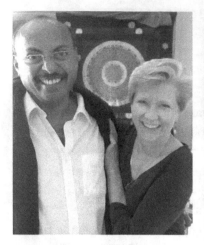 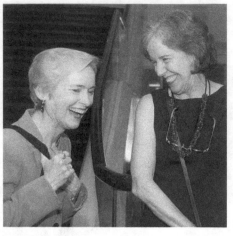

Vinoj and Ann, 2018

Reminiscing with Jane (right) about our time in Nsona Mpangu, 2015. © MARGOT I. SCHULMAN

Ann, Barbara, and Mary Luke, another former colleague, provided helpful feedback on the chapter about Ipas. I am especially indebted to Barbara who read versions of other chapters as well. I always welcomed her comments. Barbara and Mary are much better photographers than I am and provided some wonderful photos, as did Vinoj Manning who checked my references to India, too. I am extremely grateful for the many years of friendship we have all shared. A big thanks also to Terry and my siblings who reviewed relevant chapters.

Jane Bertrand, another long-time friend and colleague, confirmed my account of the memorable experience we shared 40 years ago in Zaire/DRC. In addition, she provided valuable references from her own book-writing experience. I highly recommend her 2018 book *You Started WHAT after 60? Highpointing across America.*

Neill McKee, author of the fascinating book *Finding Myself in Borneo: Sojourns in Sabah*, was also helpful in providing tips about the publishing process and sharing resources.

I was fortunate to have the assistance of an excellent copy editor, Karen Barrett-Wilt, from whom I learned a lot. It was delightful to work with her. We discovered that we shared some common interests and experiences, including living in England in our youth and studying in Florence during college.

Sara DeHaan did a terrific job on the cover and interior design of the book. I am impressed with her creativity and wide-ranging skills and experience. She manages to juggle a heavy workload efficiently and effectively while responding to the needs of her clients.

Finally, I am indebted to Terry who has always shouldered far more than his share of work on the home front, including while I wrote this book. I am particularly grateful for all the love and support he provided throughout my international career and for the unforgettable times we have experienced in France and in other travels around the world during our five decades together. We are looking forward to celebrating our golden wedding anniversary at the end of 2020, a milestone we find hard to believe we've reached!

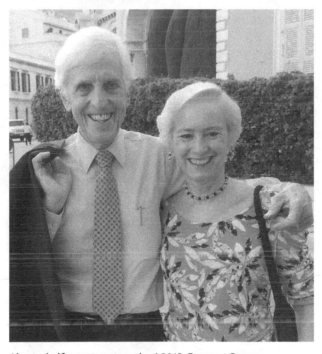

Almost half a century together! 2018. BARBARA CRANE

About the Author

Elizabeth (Liz) Maguire worked for 45 years in the international sexual and reproductive health and rights (SRHR) field, holding senior leadership positions in the U.S. government and the non-profit sector. Her multiple awards include USAID's *Distinguished Career Service Award*, the Population Institute's *Lifetime Achievement Award*, and the *Carl S. Shultz Award for Lifetime Achievement* from the American Public Health Association. In retirement, she serves as a senior SRHR advisor, dedicated to mentoring the next generation of leaders. Maguire received an M.A. in Sociology and Demography from Georgetown University. A multilingual U.S. and Irish citizen, she has lived in England, France, and Italy, and has travelled to 85 countries. Maguire currently divides her time between Chapel Hill, North Carolina and Nice, France.

CPSIA information can be obtained
at www.ICGtesting.com
Printed in the USA
LVHW090926271120
672449LV00004BA/307

9 780578 733913